Javalution

Fitness and Weight Loss Through Functional Coffee

Jose Antonio, Ph.D. & Carla Sanchez, C.S.C.S.

T0273439

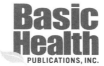

Basic Health
Health
PUBLICATIONS, INC.

The information contained in this book is based upon the research and personal and professional experiences of the authors. It is not intended as a substitute for consulting with your physician or other healthcare provider. Any attempt to diagnose and treat an illness should be done under the direction of a healthcare professional.

The publisher does not advocate the use of any particular healthcare protocol but believes the information in this book should be available to the public. The publisher and authors are not responsible for any adverse effects or consequences resulting from the use of the suggestions, preparations, or procedures discussed in this book. Should the reader have any questions concerning the appropriateness of any procedures or preparation mentioned, the authors and the publisher strongly suggest consulting a professional healthcare advisor.

Basic Health Publications, Inc.
28812 Top of the World Drive
Laguna Beach, CA 92651
949-715-7327

Library of Congress Cataloging-in-Publication Data

Antonio, Jose, Ph.D.
    Javalution : fitness and weight loss through functional coffee /
Jose Antonio & Carla Sanchez.
       p. cm.
    Includes bibliographical references and index.
    ISBN-13: 978-1-59120-169-4
    1. Coffee—Health aspects. 2. Functional foods. 3. Dietary supplements.
4. Weight loss. I. Sanchez, Carla. II. Title.

    RM246.A58   2005
    613.2—dc22

                                                    2005015023

Editor: Jane E. Morrill
Book Design and Typesetting: Gary A. Rosenberg
Cover Design by the Alison Group, Miami, FL

Printed in the United States of America

10   9   8   7   6   5   4   3   2   1

Contents

Introduction

As you read *Javalution: Fitness and Weight Loss Through Functional Coffee,* keep these points in mind:

1 ▶ Coffee is good for you.

2 ▶ Caffeine is good for you.

3 ▶ The benefits of coffee are enhanced when specific nutraceuticals are added to the blend. This type of coffee is known as "functional coffee."

4 ▶ "Everything in moderation."

Once you understand these four points, you'll be well on your way to joining the Javalution™!

Enjoy the journey. . . .

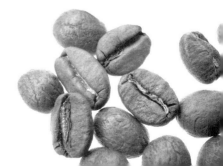

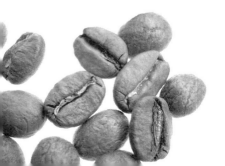

Coffee—The Magical Brown Elixir

One hundred ten million Americans can't all be wrong. That's how many coffee consumers there are in the United States. The National Coffee Association found in 2000 that 54 percent of the adult population of the United States drinks coffee daily.[1] There's a reason why millions of us wake up, rub our eyes, and plod our aching bodies to the coffeepot, take out two scoops of the brown aromatic grind, dutifully pour water in the brewer, and wait impatiently for the coffee to appear in our cups. It's because we love the taste, the aroma, and the eye-opening effects of coffee.

Coffee is good for your health. It charges up your brain. It makes exercise easier. And, to top it off, it can even help you burn fat. So, why haven't you joined the Javalution?

FUNCTIONAL COFFEE

Not only can you get the benefits of drinking coffee, which include a lower risk of type 2 diabetes and an energetic boost to your gray matter, but with the addition of "nutraceuticals" to coffee, The Javalution Coffee Company, Inc. has enhanced the health- and fitness-promoting effects of coffee. The best beverage in the world has been improved! Some food experts call this new category "functional coffee."

Let's look at functional coffee and answer some questions about it.

Is there a functional coffee that can help you lose weight?

The functional coffee JavaFit™ Burn Extreme appears to aid in weight loss. One pilot study has been conducted, and five clinical trials are in progress on this product's ability to assist in weight loss. (See Chapter 2 for more details.)

Is there a functional coffee that can give you a boost of energy?

Yes, there's a blend, JavaFit Energy Extreme, which gives you that extra boost to make running, swimming, or lifting weights feel easier. A recent study from Baylor University showed that JavaFit Energy Extreme increased resting metabolic rate (RMR) by 14.4 percent while an equal amount of Folgers coffee resulted in a decrease in metabolic rate of 5.7 percent from the pre to three-hour-post time point.

Is there a functional coffee that can help you meet your daily requirements for calcium?

The functional coffee JavaFit Lean gives you a substantial serving of calcium in your cup of coffee. A 12-ounce serving of JavaFit Lean provides approximately 110 milligrams (mg) of calcium.

Is there a functional coffee that contains vitamins and minerals?

Yes, JavaFit Complete contains approximately 50 percent or more of the daily requirements for most major vitamins and minerals. Look for JavaFit Complete to appear at your local retailer in 2006.

▶ Is there a functional coffee that contains heart-healthy ingredients?

Yes, JavaFit Heart contains folic acid and vitamins B_6 and B_{12}. Consuming sufficient quantities of these vitamins may decrease your risk of heart disease.

Coffee is the perfect delivery vehicle for many nutraceuticals. Whether it's for weight loss, energy, vitamins, minerals, or just good health, Javalution's functional coffee is one of your best tools for achieving and maintaining a healthy lifestyle.

CAFFEINE

You can't possibly discuss coffee without mentioning caffeine. In fact, caffeine and coffee are often synonymous, although this is not really the case. Caffeine is perhaps one of the most versatile ingredients known. It increases your mental alertness and ability, helps you burn fat, makes exercise seem easier, decreases your perception of pain (which is why you find it in so many pain relievers), and just plain makes you feel good. Bottom line: When used properly, caffeine is one of the things your body can really use effectively.

Caffeine, the Fat Burner

Perhaps more than any other reason, many people like to consume caffeine, whether it's in a pill or in a cup of Java, to boost their metabolism and, hence, burn more fat. Figure 1.1 illustrates the findings of several studies that show how "thermogenic" (boosting your body's metabolic rate) caffeine and coffee can be.

Note: The effects of thermogenesis on metabolism are dose- and time-dependent. In other words, the more you take, the

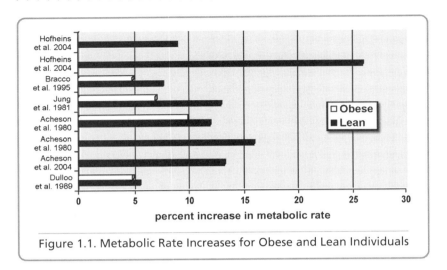

Figure 1.1. Metabolic Rate Increases for Obese and Lean Individuals

greater the effect is.[2-5] In general, you can get a significant eleva-
tion in your RMR, ranging from 5 to 30 percent, after consuming
coffee or caffeine.

Caffeine, the Brain Booster

Caffeine can work just as well as—actually better than—the
prescription medication Modafinil, which is used to improve
wakefulness in patients with the excessive daytime sleepiness
associated with narcolepsy.[6] But which is better, drinking a few
cups of Java or swallowing prescription medications that may
have unpleasant side effects? That's a no-brainer!

Here's an interesting comparative study of the two. Scientists took fifty healthy young adults and had them stay awake
for 54.5 hours! A ten-minute "vigilance test" was administered
every two hours from 8:00 A.M. on day 1 until 10:00 P.M. on day
2. At 11:55 P.M. on day 2, after 41.5 hours of being awake, double-
blind administration of one of five drug doses (placebo;
Modafinil 100, 200, or 400 mg; or caffeine 600 mg) was followed

by hourly testing. They found that 400-mg Modafinil alleviated fatigue in a manner comparable to that seen with 600 mg of caffeine. The authors concluded that the "time-on-task effects contributed to the performance degradation seen during sleep deprivation, effects [that] were reversed by caffeine and, at appropriate doses, by Modafinil."

Caffeine, the Exercise Enhancer

Dr. David Costill was the first to prove the benefits of caffeine during exercise. If you look at Figure 1.2, his study showed that the caffeine-supplemented group lasted 90.2 minutes on a bike-endurance test versus 75.5 minutes for the decaffeinated group.

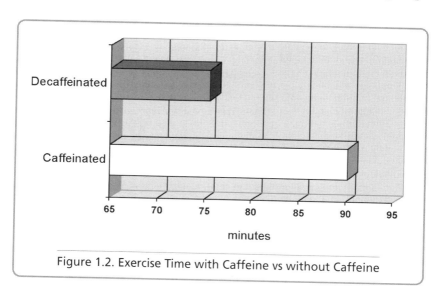

Figure 1.2. Exercise Time with Caffeine vs without Caffeine

The caffeine group also had enhanced fat-burning effects as seen in Figure 1.3. So, to summarize this landmark study: Caffeine helps you exercise longer; the exercise feels easier; and you burn more fat while doing it.

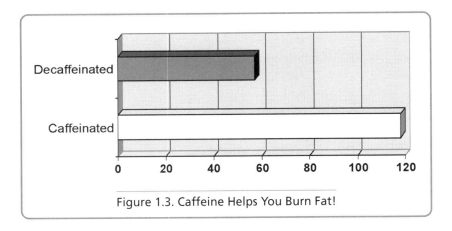

Figure 1.3. Caffeine Helps You Burn Fat!

NO NEW BEHAVIORS NEEDED

Almost anything that you can take in a pill, you can also put in functional coffee. That's the beauty of JavaFit functional coffee. How many times have you embarked on a new fad diet or novel exercise scheme? Do you even remember? Why do individuals typically quit their new-and-improved diet and exercise regimens? Because these plans require learning and maintaining new behaviors.

That's the beauty of JavaFit. If you already drink coffee, why not drink a coffee that has more benefits? So, if you're already drinking coffee, there is no need to learn a new behavior! Javalution has taken the benefits of coffee and further enhanced them—period!

2

JavaFit—
The World's First
Functional Gourmet Coffee

Tired of taking countless pills? If you open up your kitchen cabinet, you probably have calcium pills, vitamin tablets, and assorted other capsules. Then there are the various diet pills that require you to take six King Kong–sized capsules throughout the day. Who needs all that?

If you don't mind taking pills, you can skip this lecture. But if you're among the millions of Americans who want to get some of these nutrients without worrying about whether you took your pills, then here's your solution.

What if you could get the benefits of dietary supplements without changing a single behavior? In other words, you would not have to swallow extra pills, buy newfangled exercise equipment from a hyperactive spokesman on a late-night infomercial, or decipher complicated directions on the back of a label to figure out how to use it. Imagine, instead, brewing your normal cup of coffee in the morning, smelling the glorious aroma, and drinking a liquid brew that is chock full of nutrients. Sound good? Well, it's now a reality.

JavaFit from the Javalution Coffee Company is the first functional coffee to deliver the benefits of nutraceuticals in a delicious cup of gourmet coffee. There's no need to change any daily behaviors. If you already drink coffee, you can derive the benefits of functional coffee by merely switching the brand you put in the filter basket.

SCIENCE SAYS . . .
JavaFit Burn Extreme

Think about it! You can get energy supplements, weight-loss supplements, vitamins, calcium, and more just by drinking your coffee. In fact, a pilot study presented at the International Society of Sports Nutrition demonstrated how powerful functional coffee could be. Mendel, et al. examined the effect of functional coffee (JavaFit Burn Extreme) using an open-label design[1]; a total of ten healthy subjects completed two trials: ingestion of 1.5 tablespoons of coffee brewed in 12 ounces of water, and on a separate day, 2 tablespoons of coffee brewed in 12 ounces of water. Each tablespoon of the coffee contained 4.4 grams (g) of Arabica beans (ground) and 670 milligrams (mg) of a combination of *Garcinia cambogia* extract , *Citrus aurantium* extract, caffeine, and chromium polynicotinate. Compared to baseline, no harmful changes in heart rate, blood pressure, or electrocardiogram (ECG) were detected; however, resting metabolic rate (RMR) increased on average by approximately 8.9 percent and 25.6 percent after 1.5 and 2 tablespoons of brewed coffee, respectively (see Figure 2.1). According to the authors, "these data indicate that a single dose of brewed . . . JavaFit Burn Extreme . . . has dose-dependent thermogenic properties in healthy subjects."[2]

Furthermore, this group of scientists also performed an open-label trial looking at the effects of combining JavaFit Burn Extreme with exercise. They measured aspects of health and body composition in men and women. Nine healthy men and women (twenty-five to fifty-five years old with 38.4 percent body fat) ingested JavaFit Burn Extreme prior to a workout consisting of resistance exercise and aerobic exercise (cardio) over an

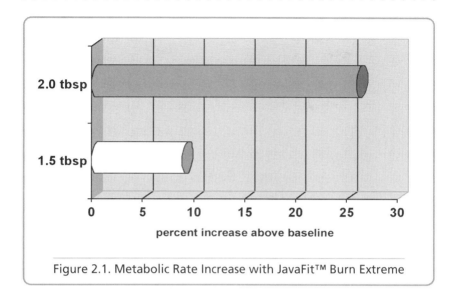

Figure 2.1. Metabolic Rate Increase with JavaFit™ Burn Extreme

eight-week treatment period. The beverage was consumed twenty to thirty minutes prior to training. Subjects were instructed to use a noncaloric sweetener or creamer, if desired; they exercised four times per week which consisted of circuit weight training followed by aerobic exercise.

The following occurred in these Java-consuming exercisers (see Figure 2.2 for changes in body composition). The subjects gained muscle and lost fat, yet their body weight didn't change. That's a good thing! It means they changed the ratio of their body to more muscle with less fat. Also, this preliminary study showed that consuming JavaFit Burn Extreme is safe. For instance, plasma glucose, or blood sugar, decreased (down 8.1 percent) as did triglycerides (down 24.4 percent). Furthermore, there was no change in total cholesterol, HDL cholesterol, or LDL cholesterol.

So, when you consume JavaFit Burn Extreme coffee prior to exercise (resistance and aerobic), it leads to positive changes in body composition. Although body weight did not change signif-

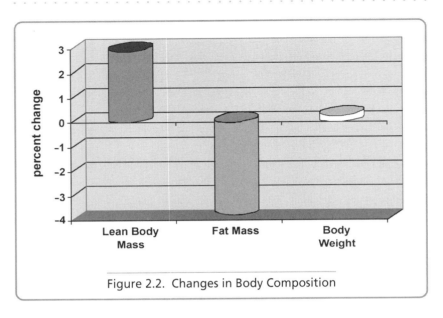

Figure 2.2. Changes in Body Composition

icantly, decreases in total percent body fat and total fat mass did occur. Also, when you look at measures of health, you'll find that cholesterol, HDL (good cholesterol), and LDL (bad cholesterol) didn't change. Furthermore, triglycerides (TAGS) and glucose decreased. Expected body-weight changes were offset by an increase in lean (muscle) mass. Ultimately, this increase in lean mass would be expected to help maintain the loss of fat mass due to an expected increase in metabolic rate (the body becomes a better calorie-burning machine).

JavaFit Energy Extreme

Not to be outdone, there was another clinical trial performed on JavaFit Energy Extreme at Baylor University (www. sportsnutrition society.org/site/conferences.php). JavaFit Energy Extreme contains additional caffeine (150 mg), green tea extract (with *Epigallocatechin gallate* [EGCG]), niacin, and *Garcinia cambogia*. JavaFit Energy Extreme was compared to regular caffeinated Folgers coffee in ten coffee-drinking subjects (five men and five women). The subjects were randomly assigned to a crossover design with the analysis separated by seven days. Resting energy expenditure (REE; kcal/day), resting heart rate (RHR), and blood pressure were performed in a supine (lying on the back) position before and one, two, and three hours after coffee ingestion. The JavaFit coffee consumption increased REE by 14.4 percent (males = 12.1 percent, females = 17.9 percent), while the Folgers coffee resulted in a decrease in REE by 5.7 percent from before to three hours after drinking the coffee. According to these investigators, "the results from this study suggest that JavaFit Energy Extreme coffee is effective at increasing REE in both male and female regular-coffee drinkers for up to three hours following the ingestion of coffee, while the ingestion of Folgers regular demonstrated no such effect." Furthermore, no adverse affects on RHR and blood pressure were found.

This is just the tip of the iceberg. Not only does Javalution have functional coffees that'll "rev up" your metabolic rate and fat-burning furnace, it has functional coffees with the health-promoting benefits of calcium, multivitamins, and more.

Making JavaFit Functional Coffee Work for You

Besides assisting you in weight management (JavaFit Burn Extreme) and giving you a boost of energy (JavaFit Energy Extreme), there are other products that can help you achieve optimal fitness, health, and wellness. For instance, JavaFit Lean with calcium can help you reach your recommended daily needs for calcium. JavaFit Complete and JavaFit Heart contain vitamins needed for normal health and those that have been shown to decrease the risk of heart disease, respectively.

METABOLISM UP—WEIGHT DOWN

With a pilot study demonstrating that JavaFit Burn Extreme can increase your metabolic rate by as much as 30 percent, it should be as clear as the Montana sky that more calories expended translates in the long haul to more weight lost. Four additional clinical trials are underway at three major universities and one clinical research organization (CRO).

Javalution has taken a great cup of coffee, made it better for you, and, to top it off, is spending thousands of dollars on research and development to ensure that it works! That's the exciting benefit of JavaFit.

3

Fat Fighter

Perhaps one of the most ridiculous things we've ever heard—by a personal trainer in a gym, no less—is that drinking coffee with caffeine will make you fat. That's right up there with spontaneous human combustion and body levitation. All you need to do is read the scientific literature to clear this up. To wit: Coffee/caffeine consumption is thermogenic—increases the metabolic rate—and promotes fat burning (oxidation).

One study looked at the thermic effect of caffeinated and decaffeinated coffee ingested with breakfast. A higher increase in metabolic rate was observed after consuming breakfast with caffeinated coffee than after eating breakfast with decaffeinated coffee.[1] This isn't rocket science. Basically, if you eat breakfast (and you should because it's the most important meal of the day) with a cup of caffeinated coffee, your metabolic rate (the number of calories you burn) is higher than it is if you drink decaffeinated coffee with breakfast.

There is plenty of science that shows that the general effect of caffeine throughout the entire body is to cause central nervous-system arousal (your brain is awake and alert), mobilize free fatty acids and other metabolites (you burn more fat), and possibly enhance the contractile status of muscle (your muscles work better).[2] See Figure 3.1 below for a graphic representation of how much caffeine elevates metabolism.

INCREASED METABOLIC RATE

One study from *The American Journal of Physiology* showed that caffeine ingestion raised energy expenditure by 9.5 to 11 percent (see Figure 3.1 below). The authors of this study said, "older and younger men show a similar thermogenic response to caffeine ingestion."[3] Another investigation examined the effect of an 8 milligram (mg) dose of caffeine per kilogram (kg) of body weight on thermogenesis (that's about 560 mg for a 154-pound person). The metabolic rate increased significantly during the three hours after caffeine ingestion. Although plasma (blood) glucose, insulin, and carbohydrate oxidation did not change significantly, plasma free-fatty-acid levels rose 96 percent and were accompanied by significant increases in fat oxidation during the last hour of the test.

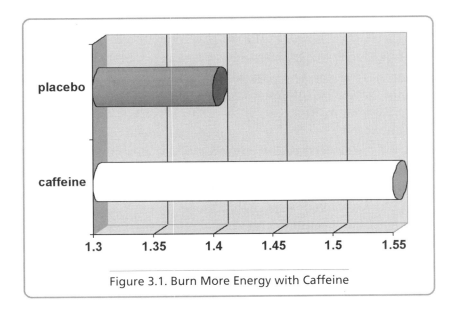

Figure 3.1. Burn More Energy with Caffeine

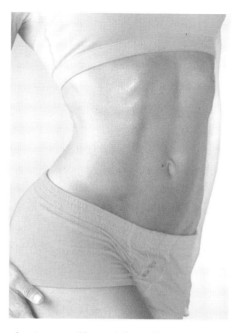

In the second and third trials, the effects of coffee providing 4 mg/kg of caffeine were studied in control and obese subjects; this is equal to about 280 mg of caffeine for a 154-pound individual. Metabolic rate increased significantly in both groups. The thermic effect of the meal was significantly greater after caffeinated coffee than after decaffeinated coffee, and, again, fat oxidation was significantly greater after caffeinated coffee. In conclusion, coffee with caffeine stimulates the metabolic rate in both control and obese individuals; however, this is accompanied by greater oxidation or burning of fat in normal-weight subjects.[4]

ERGOGENIC AID

Caffeine is one of the most famous ergogenic aids in the athletic field (that is, a drug, nutraceutical, food, or beverage that can enhance athletic performance). This was demonstrated in a clinical trial. Human subjects ingested caffeine (5 mg/kg) one hour before exercise; this is equal to 350 mg of caffeine for a 150-pound individual, or roughly three to four cups of regular coffee. The subjects exercised on a cycle ergometer at 60 percent of their VO_2 max (a measure of the maximum amount of oxygen a person can use) for forty-five minutes, and then the exercise intensity was increased to 80 percent of their VO_2 max until exhaustion. The respiratory exchange ratio (RER) of the caffeine trial was significantly lower than that of the placebo trial, indicating greater burning of fat as a fuel with caffeine. Also, endurance time to exhaustion was significantly increased after consuming caffeine. This study shows that caffeine promotes the breakdown of fat (so that it can be used as a fuel for your body), and this may, in turn, spare the amount of muscle glycogen—the stored carbohydrate energy in muscle—you use during exercise.[5]

What about age? Is there a difference between how younger and older individuals metabolize caffeine? This question was answered in a study of ten younger (aged nineteen to twenty-six) and older (aged sixty-five to eighty) men. They found that caffeine is absorbed just as well by both old and young men. But caffeine ingestion increased fatty-acid concentrations and tended to increase the rate at which fatty acids appeared in younger, but not older, men. So, in essence, while younger and older men show a similar thermogenic response (metabolic rate increase) to caffeine ingestion, older men show a smaller increase in fatty-acid availability after a caffeine challenge. This suggests that younger individuals may be better at oxidizing fat after consuming caffeine.[6]

NOT FAT—THIN!

There is convincing evidence that caffeine promotes lipolysis (the breakdown of fat) and improves exercise performance. The notion that consuming coffee or caffeine will make you fat is completely absurd. In fact, as an aid in helping to burn fat, caffeine (and perhaps other ingredients, such as green tea and "bitter orange") may serve as an effective tool in the quest for a better, fitter body.

4

Brain and Body Fuel

What's the first thing you do when you get up in the morning? If you're like many of us, you head straight for the coffeepot and make yourself a good-tasting cup or two of Java. Caffeinated coffee jumpstarts the brain from 0 to 60 faster than just about anything else. The effects of caffeine, especially caffeinated coffee, on human mental performance have been extensively studied. For example, consuming caffeinated beverages may maintain aspects of "cognitive and psychomotor performance throughout the day and evening when caffeinated beverages are administered repeatedly."[1]

One investigation examined the association of caffeinated and decaffeinated coffee intake with cognitive function in a community-based sample of older adults from 1988 to 1992. The participants were 890 women with a mean age of 72.6 years and 638 men with a mean age of 73.3 years from the Rancho Bernardo Study. Cognitive function was assessed by twelve standardized tests, and lifetime and current coffee consumption were obtained by questionnaire. Higher lifetime coffee consumption in women was associated with better performance on six of twelve mental-function tests. Lifetime and current exposure to caffeine may be associated with better cognitive performance among women, especially those aged eighty or more years.[2]

FUEL FOR MUSCLES

Caffeine is the most commonly consumed drug in the world, and athletes frequently use it as an ergogenic aid. It improves performance and endurance during prolonged, exhaustive exercise. To a lesser degree it also enhances short-term, high-intensity athletic performance. Caffeine improves concentration, reduces fatigue, and enhances alertness. Habitual intake does not diminish caffeine's ergogenic properties. Furthermore, the mechanisms of its action are not entirely understood. However, it *is* safe and does *not* cause significant dehydration or electrolyte imbalance during exercise.[3] If that doesn't make you reach for a cup-a-Joe, here's some proof that caffeine and coffee can indeed convert your body from a Volkswagon bug to high-performance race car.

In a recent study, scientists examined whether the previous drinking of caffeinated coffee (COF) decreased the ergogenic effect of the subsequent consumption of anhydrous (pill form) caffeine (CAF). Thirteen subjects performed six rides to exhaustion at 80 percent of VO_2 max ninety minutes after taking combinations of COF, decaffeinated coffee (DECAF), CAF, or placebo. The conditions were as follows:

A. DECAF + placebo (white bar in Figure 4.1)

B. DECAF + CAF (5 milligrams [mg] per kilogram [kg] of body weight)

C. COF (*1.1 mg/kg caffeine) + CAF (5 mg/kg)

D. COF (*1.1 mg/kg caffeine) + CAF (3 mg/kg)

E. COF (*1.1 mg/kg caffeine) + CAF (7 mg/kg)

F. colored water + CAF (5 mg/kg)

* This represents the dose of caffeine that subjects received from the coffee.

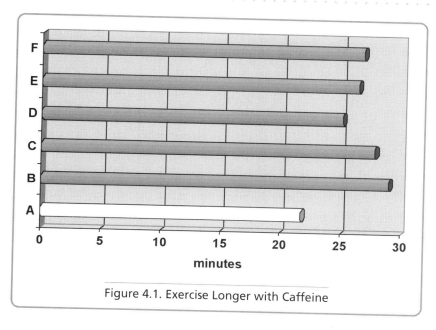

Figure 4.1. Exercise Longer with Caffeine

Times to exhaustion, as shown in Figure 4.1, were significantly greater for all trials with CAF versus placebo (trial A). Exercise times (in minutes) were:

A. 21.7 min +/− 8.1 min

B. 29.0 min +/− 7.4 min

C. 27.8 min +/− 10.8 min

D. 25.1 min +/− 7.9 min

E. 26.4 min +/− 8.0 min

F. 26.8 min +/− 8.1 min

According to the investigators, "the prior consumption of COF did not decrease the ergogenic effect of the subsequent ingestion of anhydrous CAF."[4]

Investigators also examined the effect of caffeine ingestion on work output at various levels of perceived exertion during thirty minutes of isokinetic variable-resistance cycling exercise. Ten subjects completed six trials sixty minutes after consuming either 6 mg/kg (three trials) or a placebo (three trials). This translates into 420 mg of caffeine for a 154-pound individual. Total work performed during the caffeine trials averaged 277.8 kJoules (kJ), whereas the mean total work during the placebo trials was 246.7 kJ. In other words, consuming caffeine makes exercise feel easier, so you can do more of it. In conclusion, caffeine can alter neural perception of effort significantly.[5]

Also, consuming caffeinated coffee decreases the time required to run 1,500 meters (also known as the "metric mile") and increases the speed of the "finishing burst" (also known as the "final kick") at the end of the race. Thus, caffeinated coffee is a very effective performance-enhancer.[6]

CLASSIC CAFFEINE/COFFEE STUDY

To determine what effects caffeine ingestion has on metabolism and performance during prolonged exercise, nine competitive cyclists (two females and seven males) exercised until exhaustion on a bicycle ergometer at 80 percent of VO_2 max. One test was performed an hour after drinking decaffeinated coffee (Trial D), while a second test (Trial C) required that each subject consume coffee containing 330 mg of caffeine sixty minutes before the exercise. The caffeine group lasted 90.2 minutes on the bike versus 75.5 minutes for the decaffeinated group (see Figure 1.2 on page 7).

The caffeine group also had increased fat-burning effects. Calculations of carbohydrate (CHO) metabolism from respiratory exchange ratio (RER) data revealed that the subjects oxidized, or burned, roughly 240 grams (g) of CHO in each of the two trials. But for fat burning, as shown in Figure 4.2, the caffeine group did much better (118 g or 1.31 g/min) than the decaffeinated group (57 g or 0.75 g/min). Another interesting find was that exercise "felt" easier (called the "perceived exertion rating") after drinking caffeinated coffee than it did after consuming decaf. So, caffeine helps you exercise longer; the exercise feels easier; and you burn more fat doing it.[7]

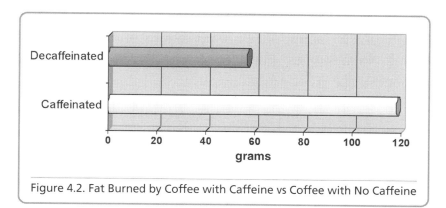

Figure 4.2. Fat Burned by Coffee with Caffeine vs Coffee with No Caffeine

Not Just For Runners

Certainly, caffeine is a great ergogenic aid for runners and cyclists. But what about athletes who carry a bit more muscle in their upper body? To answer that question, eight competitive oarswomen performed three simulated 2,000 meter (m) time trials on a rowing ergometer. The trials, which were preceded by a twenty-four-hour dietary and training control regimen and seventy-two hours of abstinence from caffeine, were conducted one hour after consuming caffeine (at 6 mg/kg or 9 mg/kg) or a

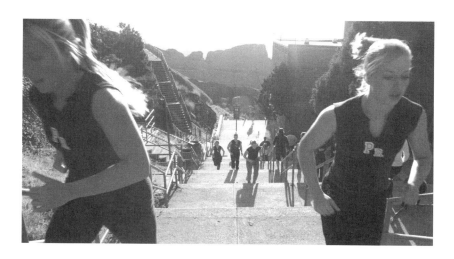

placebo. Plasma free-fatty-acid concentrations before exercise were higher with caffeine than with the placebo, suggesting that caffeine can promote the breakdown of fat. Performance time improved 0.7 percent with 6 mg/kg dose of caffeine and 1.3 percent with 9 mg/kg dose of caffeine. The first 500 m was faster with the higher caffeine dose than with the placebo or the lower dose (1.53 min versus 1.55 min and 1.56 min). Thus, caffeine enhances rowing performance mainly by improving the first 500 m of a 2,000 m row.[8]

But do you need that high a dose to achieve a performance benefit (630 mg for a 154-pound person)? Actually, you can get away with less than half that. For instance, maximal anaerobic power increases significantly after consuming only 250 mg of caffeine.

Muscle Men

Twenty elite male athletes underwent computerized testing to determine the effect of 7 mg/kg of caffeine on the strength and power of the knee extensors and flexors (quadriceps and hamstring muscles). That dose is equal to 636 mg of caffeine for a 200-

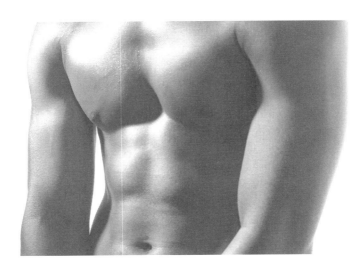

pound guy. Peak torque (T) was measured for knee extension (ET) and flexion (FT) at angular velocities of 30 degrees, 150 degrees, and 300 degrees per second. In other words, muscular power was measured at slow, medium, and fast speeds of movement. The study found significant caffeine-related increases in ET and FT at both fast and slow speeds of movement. No significant effects were found in any variable for the placebo trial. According to the authors, "it was concluded that caffeine can favorably affect some strength parameters in highly resistance-trained males."[9]

Caffeine and Sprint Swimming

Seven trained and seven untrained subjects swam freestyle for two 100-m distances, at maximum speed, separated by twenty minutes of passive recovery, once after caffeine (250 mg) and once after placebo ingestion. Only the trained subjects swam faster during the caffeine trial. This is further evidence that caffeine is not just for the endurance athlete.[10]

Pain Free

Ever wondered why many over-the-counter pain medications have caffeine added to them? Adding caffeine to aspirin and acetaminophen makes them relieve headache pain about 40 percent better than they do without it. Caffeine also helps your body absorb these medications, allowing you to get back to your daily life faster.[11, 12]

In a study, low caffeine–consuming college-aged males took one of two doses of caffeine (5 mg/kg or 10 mg/kg) or a placebo and one hour later completed thirty minutes of moderate-intensity cycling exercise (60 percent of VO_2 peak). Caffeine increased the resting systolic pressure in a dose-dependent fashion, but these blood-pressure effects were not maintained during exercise. Caffeine had a significant linear effect on leg-muscle pain ratings (the higher the dose, the better the pain relief provided by the caffeine). The average pain-intensity scores during exercise after consuming 10 mg/kg of caffeine, 5 mg/kg of caffeine, and placebo were 2.1, 2.6, and 3.5, respectively (the lower the number, the more pain relief). This is shown graphically in Figure 4.3. According to the authors, "the results support the conclusion that caffeine ingestion has a dose-response effect on reducing leg-muscle pain during exercise and that these effects do not depend on caffeine-induced increases in systolic blood pressure during exercise."[13, 14]

Both Users and Nonusers Benefit

Does the ergogenic response differ between users and nonusers of caffeine? Twenty-one subjects (thirteen caffeine users and eight nonusers) completed six randomized exercise rides to exhaustion at 80 percent of VO_2 max after ingesting either a placebo or 5 mg/kg of caffeine. Exercise to exhaustion was completed once a week at one, three, or six hours after ingestion.

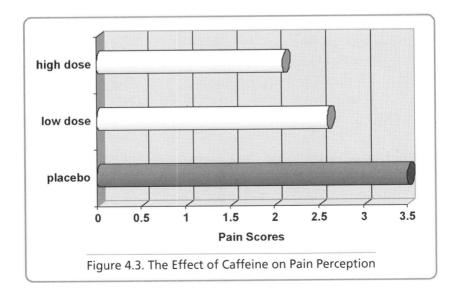

Figure 4.3. The Effect of Caffeine on Pain Perception

Exercise time to exhaustion differed between users and nonusers with the ergogenic effect being greater and lasting longer in nonusers.

For the nonusers, the exercise times at one, three, and six hours after caffeine ingestion were 32.7, 32.1, and 31.7 minutes, respectively, and these values were significantly greater than the corresponding placebo values of 24.2, 25.8, and 23.2 minutes. For caffeine users, exercise times at one, three, and six hours after caffeine ingestion were 27.4, 28.1, and 24.5 minutes, respectively. Only exercise times at one and three hours after caffeine ingestion were significantly greater than the respective placebo trials of 23.3, 23.2, and 23.5 minutes. Therefore, both users and nonusers respond positively to taking caffeine; however, nonusers may have a better ergogenic effect.[15]

Caffeine Does Not Dehydrate

According to the scientific literature, caffeine consumption stimulates a mild diuresis similar to water, but there is no evidence of a fluid-electrolyte imbalance that is detrimental to exercise performance or health. Investigations comparing caffeine (100–680 mg) to water or placebo have rarely found a statistical difference in urine volume.

In the ten studies reviewed, consumption of a caffeinated beverage resulted in 0 to 84 percent retention of the initial volume ingested, whereas consumption of water resulted in 0 to 81 percent retention. Further, tolerance to caffeine reduces the likelihood that a detrimental fluid-electrolyte imbalance will occur. Thus, athletes and recreational enthusiasts will not incur detrimental fluid-electrolyte imbalances if they consume caffeinated beverages in moderation and eat a typical American diet. What about couch potatoes? Well they'd actually have an even lower risk of dehydration because they don't exercise as hard or as long.[16]

A WONDER DRUG

If caffeine were discovered today, it would certainly be the wonder drug of the twenty-first century. It can decrease pain, improve exercise performance, and improve mental function. Is there anything else quite like it? We think not. Unfortunately, there are many myths promulgated about caffeine that we have found it necessary to dispel. There is no single ingredient or supplement on the market that provides the benefits for your brain and body that caffeine does; creatine is, perhaps, a close second.

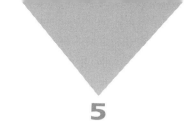

5

Health Tonic

Coffee is probably the most frequently ingested beverage worldwide (okay, second—water is the first). With such widespread consumption should come either large-scale benefits or big problems. At least that's what common sense would say. So, with billions of individuals worldwide drinking Java, we know that coffee is, in fact, a healthy beverage. And with the nutraceuticals added to JavaFit, Javalution has taken the best of coffee and made it even better.

If you're not yet convinced, read the science behind coffee's health benefits. Coffee is a very rich source of potent antioxidants. According to one study's conclusions, "it is apparent that moderate, daily, filtered coffee intake is not associated with any adverse cardiovascular effects." Quite to the contrary, the data shows that coffee has significant antioxidant activity, and even has an inverse association with the risk of type 2 diabetes.[1] Also, caffeinated coffee is a potent thermogen that is often studied by scientists for its effects on metabolic rate and fat burning.

DECREASED DIABETES RISK

One thing is certain. Coffee is perhaps one of the best health tonics available to decrease the risk of type 2 diabetes. In fact, the evidence is nothing less than robust![2-20] According to van Dam, et al. and other scientists, habitual coffee consumption is associated with higher insulin sensitivity (which is good) and a lower risk of type 2 diabetes.[21-26]

Here's the proof. In a large-scale study, 7,949 healthy Swedish subjects aged thirty-five to fifty-six years were studied. Information regarding coffee consumption and other factors was obtained by questionnaire. In subjects with type 2 diabetes and impaired glucose tolerance, high coffee consumption (five cups or more daily) was inversely associated with insulin resistance. This means that the more coffee they drank, the better off they were in regard to insulin metabolism. Scientists concluded, "the results of this study indicated that high consumers of coffee have a reduced risk of type 2 diabetes and impaired glucose tolerance. The beneficial effects may involve both improved insulin sensitivity and enhanced insulin response."[27]

In a study of a random population sample of 1,361 Swedish women, scientists found the risk of developing diabetes was 475 per 100,000 person-years in women who consumed two cups of coffee or less per day, 271 per 100,000 person-years in women who consumed three to four cups per day, 202 with a consumption of five to six cups per day, and 267 in drinkers of seven cups or more per day.[28] So, it looks like consuming as many as six cups of coffee per day actually has a *protective* effect against diabetes!

Another large-scale study, the Nurses' Health Study and Health Professionals' Follow-up Study, followed 41,934 men from 1986 to 1998 and 84,276 women from 1980 to 1998. These participants did not have diabetes, cancer, or cardiovascular disease at the beginning of the study. They found an inverse association between coffee intake and type 2 diabetes after adjusting for age, body mass index (BMI), and other risk factors. To put it another way, the more coffee they drank, the less chance they had of getting type 2 diabetes. Total caffeine intake from coffee and other sources was associated with a statistically significant lower risk of diabetes in both men and women.[29]

Clearly, one benefit of drinking coffee is a drop in the risk of diabetes. This is significant since diabetes is the fifth leading cause of death by disease in the United States.[30] Diabetics are also at higher risk for heart disease, blindness, kidney failure, extremity amputations, and other chronic conditions. Direct medical and indirect expenditures attributable to diabetes in 2002 were estimated at $132,000,000,000 (that's 132 *billion* U.S. dollars). Healthcare spending in 2002 for people with diabetes was more than double the spending for those without the disease. Furthermore, the burden imposed by diabetes is a substantial cost to society and, in particular, to those individuals with diabetes and their families.[31]

DECREASED RISK OF CANCER

As impressive as the data is regarding coffee and diabetes, there is equally impressive data to suggest that regular coffee consumption may decrease the risk of certain cancers. Caffeinated (not decaffeinated) coffee may decrease the risk of oral/pharyngeal and esophageal cancer.[32] Interestingly, this is not true of tea. There is also very recent data on liver cancer (hepatocellular carcinoma [HCC]) and coffee. Frequent coffee intake was significantly associated in an inverse relation to HCC mortality in both men and women with a history of liver disease.[33]

A study of more than 90,000 Japanese found that a protective effect occurred in people who drank one to two cups of coffee a day and that the protection increased at three to four cups a day. The likely occurrence of liver cancer in people who never, or almost never, drank coffee was 547.2 cases per 100,000 people over ten years.[34] On the other hand, among those who drank coffee daily, the risk was 214.6 cases per 100,000. The study also looked at green tea and found no such association between drinking green tea and liver cancer rates.

Women with epithelial ovarian cancer (EOC) showed an inverse relationship between caffeine intake and EOC, but tea consumption was not related to EOC. Translation: Drinking more coffee seems to benefit those with EOC. This isn't a caffeine-related issue, per se, because tea didn't have a similar effect. As tea contributed significantly to caffeine intake in this population, scientists concluded that the "association we observed with coffee is not due to caffeine, but to other components within coffee."[35] Moreover, colon cancer risk is inversely associated with drinking coffee.[36]

There are, of course, many other types of cancer. In addition to decreasing the risk of colon, ovarian, liver, and oral/pharyngeal cancer, coffee has also been proven safe in relation to some other types of cancer. In a study of Swedish women, consumption of coffee, tea, and caffeine were not associated with the incidence of breast cancer.[37] And there is no association between coffee intake and the risk of pancreatic cancer.[38]

HEART DISEASE

There is a popular misconception that coffee increases your risk of heart problems. It's not true. Large prospective studies do not support the hypothesis that moderate (two to four cups of coffee per day) caffeine consumption significantly increases the risk of coronary heart disease.[39] Also, according to the *Journal of Clinical Hypertension,* even being a coffee drinker for thirty-three years is not associated with developing hypertension.[40]

Specifically, here's the data. Scientists observed 1,935 patients who were hospitalized with a confirmed acute myocardial infarction between 1989 and 1994 at forty-five community hospitals and tertiary-care centers in the United States, as part of the Determinants of Myocardial Infarction Onset Study. The scientists found that coffee consumption was not associated with an overall change in the long-term post-infarction mortality rate; in other words, it had no effect on the death rate.[41]

In Croatia, death rates are higher than those in the countries of the European Union (EU) and consumption of coffee is moderate compared to that in EU countries. Data was obtained from an epidemiological longitudinal study that was started in 1969, with follow-ups in 1972—including 1,571 men and 1,793 women aged thirty-five to fifty-nine years—and 1982—including 1,093 men and 1,330 women. The study found no significant effects of coffee consumption on general mortality and mortality due to cardiovascular disease among men.

Positive effects of coffee on general mortality but not on cardiovascular disease–associated mortality were observed among women. Women who regularly drank one to two cups of coffee per day had a significantly lower risk of death from all causes, adjusted for age, region, smoking, diastolic blood pressure, feeling of well-being, and history of stomach ulcer.[42] In other words, drinking moderate amounts of coffee had no effect on cardiovascular disease risk in men or women. But general mortality was lower in women who drank coffee.

A very large-scale study examined female registered nurses in the United States, a total of 85,747 American women aged thirty-four to fifty-nine years in 1980 with no history of coronary heart disease (CHD), stroke, or cancer. The ten-year incidence of CHD (defined as nonfatal myocardial infarction or fatal CHD) was assessed. They found no association on CHD with caffeine intake from all sources combined or with consumption of decaffeinated coffee. Scientists concluded that "coffee as consumed by U.S. women is not an important cause of CHD."[43]

A study cohort of 20,179 randomly selected eastern Finnish men and women aged thirty to fifty-nine years to participate in a cross-sectional risk-factor survey in 1972, 1977, or 1982. Habitual coffee drinking, health behavior, major known CHD risk factors, and medical history were assessed at the baseline examination. Each subject was followed for ten years after the survey using the national hospital discharge and death registers. In men, the risk of nonfatal myocardial infarction was not associated with coffee drinking. *Interestingly, the highest CHD mortality was found among those who did not drink coffee at all.* In women, all-cause mortality decreased by increasing coffee drinking. Thus, this study provides more evidence that drinking coffee does not increase the risk of CHD or death.[44]

BLOOD PRESSURE

A study was done of 3,336 male Japanese self-defense officials aged forty-eight to fifty-six years, who received a pre-retirement health examination at the Self-Defense Forces Fukuoka Hospital between October 1986 and December 1992. Average coffee intake in the previous year was ascertained by a self-administered questionnaire. They discovered that regular coffee drinkers had lower blood pressure than nondrinkers at any level of alcohol use, cigarette smoking, obesity, and glucose intolerance. The scientists concluded that this study "consolidates the previous observation that habitual coffee consumption was associated with lower blood pressure."[45]

Data on coffee consumption was collected for 1,074 adults coming in for health checks in the OXCHECK study (in the United Kingdom). Coffee had no significant effects on total or high-density lipoprotein (HDL) cholesterol or blood pressure, and was negatively correlated with serum triglycerides; in other words, the more coffee they drank, the lower the triglyceride levels became (which is good). The type of coffee consumed in the United Kingdom does not adversely affect these cardiovascular risk factors.[46]

If you have high blood pressure, it would be wise to consult with your physician. For instance, there is evidence that restriction of coffee intake may be beneficial in older hypertensive individuals.[47] Also, older middle-aged men with hypertension who consume large amounts of coffee should consider reducing their coffee intake.[48]

CHECK IT OUT

A common refrain that we often hear goes something like this: "They say that coffee is bad for you . . . gives you high blood pressure and dehydrates you . . ." We ask, who exactly is "they"? A typical response is "hmmm . . . not sure who 'they' are . . . but that's what they say." When these individuals realize how silly their statements sound, it dawns on them that perhaps all these comments about coffee or caffeine being bad for you have no basis in truth. All we ask is, read the science.

6

The Javalution Nutrition Program

Over the last two decades, American eating habits have gone from bad to deadly. According to the National Health and Nutrition Examination Survey (NHANES), more than 65 percent of all American adults are overweight. Even scarier, more than 35 percent of American adults exceed their ideal weight by at least 20 percent, earning them the dubious distinction of being "obese." How do these figures translate in terms of our health as a nation? To put it simply, nearly two-thirds of Americans are at increased risk of developing high blood pressure, diabetes, cardiovascular disease (CVD), cancer, and arthritis as a direct result of their weight. Many of these same individuals will also encounter job discrimination and social rejection, suffer from low self-esteem and depression, and die prematurely. The "human" cost of this ongoing tragedy may be incalculable, but the fiscal impact it is having on our healthcare system is unmistakably clear. If something doesn't change—and *soon*—the American lifestyle will bankrupt the American people.

NUTRITION 101: EATING FOR LOOKS AND LONGEVITY

The first step to reversing this catastrophic trend is to change our eating habits. The American diet is rich in processed foods, chemical preservatives, and artificial ingredients. Every year, we gobble more fast food, more junk food, more refined sugars and grains, and more fatty cuts of meat. Every year, our diet contains less fresh fruit, fewer vegetables, and an increasingly inadequate quantity of micronutrients. To top it all off, we are more sedentary than any other nation on Earth. With obesity on the rise at an unprecedented rate, Americans are the fattest, most inactive individuals on the entire planet, and it's killing us.

In an era when the knowledge of the ages literally exists at our fingertips, it seems ironic that we have yet to develop an efficient approach to permanent weight loss. The difficulty lies in the fact that most weight-loss programs attempt to oversimplify a complex, multifactor problem, and as a result, address the *symptoms* of weight gain rather than its underlying cause. Moreover, the vast majority of so-called "diets" cater to the American penchant for quick fixes. Unfortunately, when it comes to healthy eating, there's no such thing as a magic wand. Fad diets that eliminate entire food groups and starvation diets that severely restrict calories contradict the basic machinery of human physiology. In the long run, these approaches are doomed to fail.

Although severe caloric restriction may lead to initial weight loss, the very nature of such an approach precludes its long-term effectiveness. Weight loss by caloric restriction triggers hormonal modifications that evolved in our species so we could survive times of famine. These physiological mechanisms involve metabolic slowing, muscle catabolism (breakdown), exaggerated fat retention, and changes in brain chemistry which contribute to the development of behaviors such as binge eating. The preferential loss of lean tissue (muscle) over fat often results in a false sense of accomplishment. You *do* lose weight; however, the "new you" is merely a smaller, flabbier version of the old you. We call this being a "skinny fat."

Once normal eating patterns resume, the weight rapidly returns, plus an added ten pounds. Why? Because the muscle you sacrificed during the period of forced starvation, combined with metabolic slowing, make it that much harder for your body to burn fat. Many people will repeat this futile exercise over and over again, creating the vicious cycle of starvation and weight gain often referred to as "yo-yo dieting."

Like it or not, the only way to achieve permanent weight loss is to adopt healthy eating habits. The first step involves education. But don't panic! You won't need an advanced degree in physiology to make healthy choices about the foods that you put into your body. When you arm yourself with a fundamental understanding of macronutrients, healthy eating becomes second nature.

UNDERSTANDING BASIC NUTRIENTS

Water is vital to life. About 70 percent of the human body is comprised of water. All the chemical processes and reactions that allow us to move, breathe, think, and otherwise function as living organisms occur within an aqueous medium. Moreover, water aids with the systemic treatment and elimination of metabolic waste products.

Adequate fluid intake is especially important to active individuals seeking to improve body composition, enhance performance, or simply maximize training results. Proper hydration is needed for optimal metabolic functioning. Hence, the well-hydrated individual will

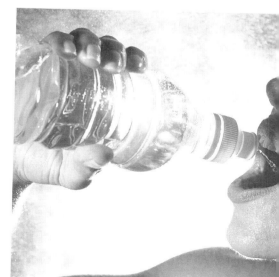

have a more comfortable and effective workout. In addition, water is also an excellent diuretic. Not only will high fluid intake increase urination, it will also decrease overall water retention and bloat. Since we do not feel thirsty until we are already in a dehydrated state, it's best to drink water in sufficient amounts and with sufficient frequency to prevent, rather than to quench, thirst.

Most sources recommend that individuals consume a minimum of two liters of water per day. If you are active, we recommend a minimum of three to four liters of water (or water-based fluids) per day. Although you may have to work up to this volume gradually over a week or so while your bladder adjusts, you will reap the benefits of your efforts almost immediately. Not only does water act as a natural appetite suppressant, but drinking water below your body temperature can actually help you to liberate calories. In fact, there is evidence to suggest that if you are well-hydrated, your body is better at burning fat.[1] If you do nothing but increase the amount of water you drink every day, you will likely notice more radiant skin, increased energy, enhanced mental focus, and greater stamina during physical exertion.

Proteins are the primary building blocks of human tissue and contain 4 calories per gram (kcal/g). Proteins are made up of complex chains of twenty different amino acids, twelve of which the body is able to manufacture. Because the human body lacks the necessary enzymes to synthesize the eight remaining amino acids from their components, these eight essential amino acids must be consumed in the diet. Protein sources that contain the full complement of essential amino acids are said to be "complete" proteins. Whole foods such as milk, cheese, eggs, poultry, meat, fish, and other seafood represent rich sources of complete protein.

In order to maintain their lean tissue mass, active individuals typically require more protein per pound of body weight per day than those who are sedentary. Power athletes, such as sprinters, football players, and individuals who engage in regular resistance training, are in a perpetual cycle of muscle breakdown and repair and demonstrate even larger protein requirements.[2–4]

Despite long-standing concerns about high-protein diets, there is not one shred of scientific evidence that increased protein intake is harmful to healthy individuals with normal kidney function.[5] Another concern that has no merit is that "high-protein" intakes contribute to bone loss. That's baloney![6–12]

Carbohydrates contain 4 kcal/g and are the main energy source for the body. For simplicity's sake, carbohydrates can be divided into two broad subcategories: fibrous carbohydrates and starchy carbohydrates.

Because fiber cannot be digested by the human gastrointestinal (GI) tract, functionally speaking, fibrous carbohydrates are calorically vacant. Fiber is, nonetheless, vital to good health. Inadequate dietary fiber leads to a sluggish GI tract, water retention, bloating, constipation, and an increased risk of developing colon cancer. In addition to being rich in vitamins, minerals, and antioxidants, fruits, vegetables, and legumes are excellent sources of fiber. You should consume a minimum of five servings of fresh fruit and vegetables every day.

Unlike fibrous carbohydrates, starchy carbohydrates are energy-dense foods that serve as a primary energy source. But all starchy carbohydrates are not created equal. During the digestive process, carbohydrates are broken down into their component sugars and absorbed through the walls of the GI tract into the bloodstream. Once in the bloodstream, they are delivered to target tissues where they are either used for immediate energy or stored as fuel for later use.

Carbohydrates are stored in the liver and muscles in the form of glycogen, which serves as the primary fuel source for muscle, especially during high-intensity exercise such as sprinting, weight training, and similar activities. Glycogen reservoirs are limited. Once the liver and muscles are saturated with glycogen, excess carbohydrate calories can "spill over" into fat stores. As little as twenty to thirty minutes of moderate-intensity aerobic activity begins to significantly deplete glycogen stores. At this point, the body will begin to dip into its fat stores for continued energy production.

The rate at which carbohydrates are broken down and absorbed into the bloodstream to induce a rise in blood sugar is quantitatively described by the glycemic index. The lower the glycemic index of a given carbohydrate, the more gradually it enters the bloodstream and, thus, the more time the body has to utilize the molecules for fuel rather than storing them as fat. Whole grains, legumes, and yams are among the best sources of low glycemic-index (LGI) carbohydrates.

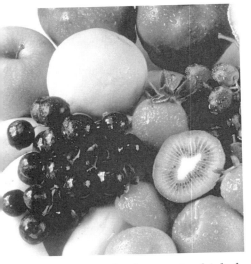

Processed foods such as white bread and white rice, and even unprocessed foods such as potatoes, have high glycemic indices (HGI) and are assimilated very rapidly. This is also true for the vast majority of simple sugars including sucrose, dextrose, lactose, and glucose. However, there is one very important exception to this rule; fructose, the sugar found in fruit, has a very low glycemic index. Due to the gradual rate at which fructose enters the bloodstream to influence insulin levels, it is unlikely to "spill over" and wind up stored as fat. You should select LGI/high-fiber carbohydrates to complete your meals throughout the day; however, HGI carbohydrates are preferred following intense exercise to enhance muscle recovery and replenish depleted glycogen stores.

Fats are an important secondary energy source, especially when muscle glycogen stores become depleted after the first twenty to thirty minutes of intense physical activity. Fats contain 9 kcal/g, more than twice the amount found in carbohydrates and proteins. Saturated fats, derived from animal sources, may contribute to the development of CVD. The healthier dietary choice is unsaturated fats, which are derived from plant sources. A balanced diet, which derives 25 to 30 percent of its total calories from fat sources, is optimal for overall health.

Alcohol is not exactly classified as a nutrient, but it is widely consumed and warrants mention. Alcohol contains 7 kcal/g so it isn't a low-calorie item by any means. However, moderate consumption of alcohol may indeed be healthy. For example, moderate intake of alcohol, including wine, is associated with a lower risk of CVD. Several investigations have reported that in "subjects consuming wine in moderation, the risk of mortality from all causes is 20 to 30 percent lower than in abstainers."[13] However, the key word is "moderation."

WHAT KINDS OF CALORIES?

Today, health-conscious individuals are well-informed about the importance of optimal body composition and are no longer as interested in just shedding pounds as they are in losing inches. They know that building muscle tissue not only improves their appearance, it also accelerates fat loss and helps make their physique goals not only attainable, but maintainable.

As the pursuit of weight loss evolves to that of improving body composition, savvy consumers want to know if, as the supplement ads claim, you can actually maintain, or even build, muscle while losing fat. Intuitively, the whole idea seems to defy logic. After all, it takes an excess of calories to build tissue and a deficit to lose tissue. Right? Wrong! Dozens of studies have demonstrated that diet and exercise can indeed lead to concurrent fat loss and lean-tissue (muscle) gain. In fact, choosing the right type of nutrients alone can improve your body composition.[14–21]

In order to understand how these two apparently contradictory processes might occur simultaneously, one must first reject certain archaic—albeit widely accepted—beliefs about human physiology. Despite half a century of research to the contrary, many people (including, unfortunately, physicians, dietitians, and nutritionists) continue to view human metabolism as a bank account into which we deposit and withdraw calories like currency. The notion that you need to "spend" more calories than you consume in order to lose body fat is not completely accurate. As scientists are learning, for lasting results in terms of fat loss and improved body composition, the *quality* of the calories you consume is more important than the overall quantity.

Protein: The Cornerstone to Permanent Fat Loss

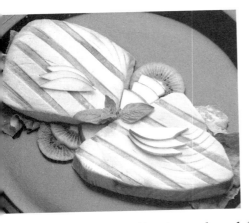

Protein is not only the building block of muscle, it is also the key to simultaneous fat loss and muscle gain. When caloric and protein consumption are adequate, dietary protein is used to construct and maintain muscle tissue. However, during times of caloric restriction, protein is converted to glucose for energy. Hence, if your fat-loss program dictates reduced fat or carbohydrate intake, your protein consumption must increase or your body will break down existing muscle to generate fuel. Just how bad is it to sacrifice a little muscle to burn fat? As it turns out, it's utterly counterproductive to your fat-loss goals!

The more muscle you have, the higher your resting metabolic rate (RMR) is and the greater your overall caloric expenditure is.[22, 23] Sedentary adults typically lose between five and seven pounds of lean muscle mass every ten years. This fact alone has enormous bearing on why people tend to gain weight as they age. Assuming your activity level and daily caloric intake remained constant over the ten years of gradual muscle loss, that adds up to a fat gain of more than fifteen pounds during the tenth year alone!

So, how much protein should you consume if you are trying to lose fat without sacrificing muscle? Your body's ability to utilize protein is closely linked to activity level. Protein requirements increase significantly if you exercise regularly. For optimal muscle retention, studies indicate that individuals who exercise regularly need approximately 1 g of protein per pound of body weight daily. If you're an average gym-goer who lifts weights two or three times a week, plus you do some form of cardiovascular exercise two or three times a week, your training makes you both an endurance and a strength athlete. In other words, if you weigh 160 pounds, you would want to eat about 160 g of protein per day. This is roughly equivalent to the amount of protein found in a half-dozen chicken breasts or five cans of tuna fish.

That's a lot of protein! Most active individuals don't consume anywhere near the amount of protein they need in order to maintain muscle tissue and prevent overtraining. And when it comes to protein, how *often* you eat is just as important as how *much* you eat. Five or six small meals and snacks per day are typically recommended for optimal fat burning and muscle retention. In order for most individuals to consume 0.75 g of protein per pound of body weight per day, they need to take in 20–30 g of protein per meal.

But what happens to the "extra calories" from increased protein intake? Can "too much" protein make you fat? Not likely! First, protein digestion requires significant energy expenditure. The thermogenesis that accompanies the consumption of a high-protein meal measurably raises your body temperature and metabolic rate. Second, due to complex hormonal relationships between glucagon and insulin, it's virtually impossible for your body to turn excess protein into glucose and store it as fat. This is the single most important governing principle behind the initial success of every high-protein diet, program, and product in existence. Notice we said "initial." The long-term viability of an eating plan—whether or not you can tolerate it over time, whether it will continue to produce the desired effects, and whether it is ultimately a healthy diet—depends largely on the two remaining macronutrients: carbohydrates and fat.

Carbohydrates: Choose Wisely!

As far as your body is concerned, all carbohydrate calories are not alike. For example, fibrous carbohydrates, which include leafy green vegetables, cauliflower, broccoli, and peppers, are essentially lacking in calories. While it's true that the carbo-

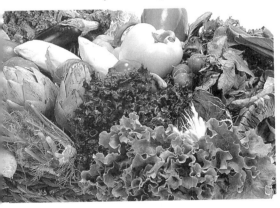

hydrates found in fiber contain 4 kcal/g just like the carbohydrates found in cookies and bread, their fibrous—rather than starchy—molecular configuration renders them virtually indigestible by humans. Fiber keeps our colons active and prevents cancer, but we can't use it as an effective energy source. You can eat as many green leafy vegetables as your heart desires, and you will never gain an ounce of fat.

As for energy-dense starchy carbohydrates, which include everything from bread to potatoes to legumes and grains, studies indicate that the glycemic index of the carbohydrate can make all the difference. The glycemic index of a food indicates the rise in blood sugar that particular food will produce over time. The glycemic index is directly related to the total number of carbohydrates the food contains, as well as the rate at which the food is digested, broken down into its component parts and absorbed through the intestinal walls into the bloodstream.

Typically, the more processed the food item is, the higher its glycemic index is, and the more rapidly it will enter the bloodstream. HGI carbohydrates, including sugary desserts and soda, fruit juice, white bread, white rice, honey, and potatoes, flood your system with glucose. The result is an energy rush caused by transient hyperglycemia (high blood sugar), which signals the pancreas to secrete a surge of insulin. The insulin surge or "spike" acts to rapidly clear glucose from your bloodstream, thereby preventing your body from burning the glucose for energy and increasing the likelihood that excess calories will wind up stored as fat. In addition, the resulting hypoglycemia (low blood sugar) can leave you feeling lethargic and hungry. There are certain times, however, that consuming HGI carbohydrates and causing an insulin surge is ideal. Immediately following high-intensity exercise or exercise lasting longer than ninety minutes, consuming HGI carbohydrates will quickly replenish muscle glycogen stores and aid in muscle recovery, without sabotaging your fat-loss efforts.

A growing amount of research indicates that consuming HGI carbohydrates can have a devastating effect on your effort to lose fat and to maintain fat loss, if not strictly limited to the time immediately following high-intensity exercise. For example, the consumption of HGI carbohydrates during a period of caloric restriction can lead to a decrease in metabolic rate and overall caloric expenditure. In addition, HGI meals have been shown to elicit a sequence of hormonal changes which decreases fat burning, contributes to overeating, and increases protein catabolism (muscle breakdown). The solution? For healthy, permanent fat loss without sacrificing muscle, eliminate processed foods and sugary drinks from your diet. Instead, choose a variety of LGI carbohydrates, such as fruits, vegetables, legumes, yams, and whole grains, to complete your meals and limit HGI carbohydrates, such as honey, rice, and potatoes, to following intense exercise only.

Fats—Go with the PUFAs and MUFAs!

PUFAs and MUFAs! Sounds like a Swedish massage. In actuality, they stand for polyunsaturated fatty acids (PUFAs) and monounsaturated fatty acids (MUFAs). In recent years, high-protein/ high-fat diets have taken the weight-loss world by storm. Although these eating plans produce rapid results early on, long-term compliance is poor. Lost in the low-versus-high-carbohydrate diet battle is the critical role played by fats. Without adequate consumption of healthy fats, you'd look like a starving chicken with no feathers. Okay, maybe not that bad, but fats (like proteins) are *necessary* for life. They are *essential* nutrients.

However, whereas low- to moderate-fat intake is good, *no* fat is *not* good! Adequate dietary fat is crucial to both good health and weight loss. Fat is not only necessary for countless physiological processes, it actually prevents overeating by contributing to a feeling of fullness. In addition, because fat slows the absorption of glucose, it helps to stabilize blood-sugar levels and reduces the likelihood that ingested carbohydrates will wind up stored as fat. However, not all fats are created equal. The types of fat you choose to include in your diet have an impact on your body composition, as well as your overall health.

▶ *Trans fats: lethal indeed*! Trans fats (TFAs) are made when manufacturers add hydrogen to vegetable oil—a process called hydrogenation. Why do food manufacturers do this? Hydrogenation increases the shelf life and flavor stability of foods containing these fats. Where can you find TFAs? Trans fats can be found in vegetable shortenings, some margarines, crackers, cookies, snack foods, and other foods made with, or fried in, partially hydrogenated oils. A small amount of trans fat is found naturally, primarily in dairy products, some meat, and other animal-based foods.[24]

Metabolic studies have clearly shown that TFAs elevate LDL and lower HDL cholesterol. Epidemiologic studies showed a relation between TFA intake and the risk of myocardial infarction (MI) or heart attack.[25]

► *Saturated fats: use sparingly*! Thus named because their chemical structure includes a full complement of hydrogen atoms at every carbon, saturated fats are solid at room temperature. Although most saturated fats you are likely to encounter are derived from animal sources, they can also be found in certain plant sources, for example, vegetable shortening. One study estimated the effects on the incidence of heart disease and associated costs of reducing dietary saturated-fat intake as a percent of total energy. They found that "reducing saturated fat intake by one to three percentage points would reduce CHD incidence by 32,000 to 99,700 events and yield combined savings in medical expenditures and lost earnings ranging from $4.1 to $12.7 billion over ten years (estimates in 1993 U.S. dollars)." Thus, reducing dietary intake of saturated fat may prevent tens of thousands of cases of heart disease and save billions of dollars in medical costs.[26] Some of the more common sources of saturated fats include fatty cuts of red meat, chicken skin, whole milk, butter, cream, and lard.

► *Unsaturated fats: substitute for saturated fats whenever possible*! Unsaturated fats are derived from plant sources and are usually liquid at room temperature but solid when refrigerated. Unsaturated-fat consumption has been shown to raise HDL (good cholesterol) levels while simultaneously lowering LDL (bad cholesterol) levels. Unsaturated fat has also been credited with reducing the risk of CVD, stroke, obesity, and diabetes. A study showed that if you want to favorably improve the LDL/HDL cholesterol ratio, changing the proportions of dietary fatty acids may be more important than restricting the percentage of total or saturated fat energy, meaning that it may be wise to replace saturated fat with a combination of MUFAs and PUFAs (rather than just decreasing the total saturated-fat intake).[27] The healthiest sources of unsaturated fat include sesame oil, soy oil, hemp oil, olives and olive oils, almonds and almond butter, and avocados.

▶ *Fish oil—the Rolls Royce of fats*! Fish oil, which contains a type of fat called the omega-3 or n-3 fatty acids, has been studied

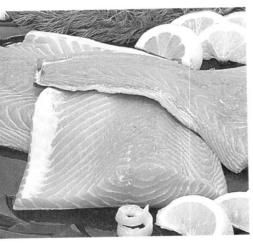

for more than thirty years. Specifically, there are two fats called docosahexaenoic and eicosapentaenoic acid that are extremely beneficial.[28] Consumption of one gram of fish oil daily has been shown to reduce overall and cardiovascular mortality, myocardial infarction, and sudden cardiac death. In addition, higher doses may be used for the ability of fish oil to lower triglycerides (fat in blood) and to reduce non-steroidal anti-inflammatory use in patients with rheumatoid arthritis. Omega-3 fatty-acid supplementation for infants has also been shown to improve infant neural growth and development. Several fish species, including sardines, mackerel, herring (Atlantic and Pacific), lake trout, salmon (Chinook, Atlantic, and Sockeye), anchovy (European), sablefish, and bluefish, provide an adequate amount of omega-3 fats and meet the nutritional recommendation of the American Heart Association (AHA).[29]

Macronutrient Manipulation

It should be as clear as distilled water that choosing the "right" macronutrients (lean proteins, healthy fats, and LGI/high-fiber carbohydrates) plays an important role in building the body you want. In fact, there is now an abundance of scientific proof which shows that by merely taking out some carbohydrates and replacing them with an equal amount of protein—with no difference in caloric intake—can improve lean body mass, promote fat loss, and enhance health.

A study compared the effects of a low-carbohydrate, ketogenic diet program with those of a low-fat, low-cholesterol, reduced-calorie diet. There were 120 overweight, hyperlipidemic (high cholesterol and triglyceride levels in the blood) volunteers from the community. The diet interventions were: 1) low-carbohydrate diet (initially, less than 20 g of carbohydrates daily) plus nutritional supplementation, exercise recommendation, and group meetings, and 2) low-fat diet (less than 30 percent energy from fat, less than 300 mg of cholesterol daily, and a deficit of 500 to 1,000 kcal/day) plus exercise recommendations and group meetings. At twenty-four weeks, weight loss was greater in the low-carbohydrate diet group than in the low-fat diet group (a mean change of 12.9 percent down vs 6.7 percent down respectively). The scientists concluded: "Compared with a low-fat diet, a low-carbohydrate diet program had better participant retention and greater weight loss. During active weight loss, serum triglyceride levels decreased more and high-density lipoprotein cholesterol level increased more with the low-carbohydrate diet than with the low-fat diet."[30]

Another study looked at the effects of a very low-carbohydrate diet on body composition and cardiovascular risk factors.[31] Subjects were randomized to six months of either a very low-carbohydrate diet or a calorie-restricted diet with 30 percent of the calories as fat. Fifty-three healthy, obese female volunteers were randomized; forty-two completed the trial. The low-carbohydrate group lost more weight (8.5 kilograms [kg] vs 3.9 kg) and more body fat (4.8 kg vs 2.0 kg).

Volek, et al. examined the effects of a six-week very low-carbohydrate diet on total and regional body composition.[32] Interestingly, their results indicated that fat mass was significantly decreased (down 3.4 kg) and lean body mass was significantly increased (up 1.1 kg) at week six.

It's the *Kind* of Calories!

How does choosing certain nutrients affect body composition? Scientists believe that the better effect of protein versus carbohydrate in enhancing body composition can be explained primarily by the enhanced thermogenesis (seen with low-carbohydrate diets).[33] The hormonal changes associated with replacing carbohydrates with an equal amount of protein include a reduction in the circulating levels of insulin. For example, a recent study demonstrated that postprandial thermogenesis—in other words, how much your metabolic rate goes up after eating—was increased 100 percent on a high-protein/low-fat diet versus a high-carbohydrate/low-fat diet in healthy subjects.[34]

Now this doesn't mean you should embark on a low-carbohydrate diet. It means that you need to find a diet that you can comply with and follow most of the time. Keep in mind that of all the food choices you can make, in general, you should consume saturated fats and HGI/low-fiber/high-sugar carbohydrates sparingly. If you follow that simple piece of advice, you'll be well on your way to a better body.

SUMMARY—NUTRITION 101

1 ▶ *Eat frequent, small meals.* For best results in terms of high energy level, diminished body fat, muscle growth and maintenance, and good GI health, you should eat five to six small meals and snacks throughout the day. The longer your body waits between meals, the less efficient it becomes at burning fat and the greater your chance of overeating when you finally feed yourself.

2 ▶ *Include protein with every meal.* Protein contains 4 kcal/g. Get approximately 1 g of protein daily per pound of body weight. In general, active individuals have higher protein requirements because they are constantly tearing down and rebuilding their muscle tissue. To promote optimal body composition—in other words, to lose fat without losing muscle—you should consume one serving (20–30 g, or 80–120 kcal) of protein with each meal. If this seems like a tall order, we highly recommend that you consider using meal-replacement powders or protein shakes to help meet your protein needs.

3 ▶ *Select high-fiber/LGI carbohydrates to complete your meals.* Limit HGI carbohydrate consumption to following high-intensity exercise only. The lower the glycemic index of a given carbohydrate, the more gradually it will be digested into its component parts and absorbed from the GI tract into the bloodstream. Less insulin is released from the pancreas over a given time in response to LGI foods. Hence, the body has more time to utilize the molecules for fuel rather than storing them as fat. Whole grains, legumes, pasta, and yams are among the best sources of complex carbohydrates. Processed foods such as white rice and bread, and even unprocessed foods such as potatoes, have higher glycemic indices, are assimilated at rates similar to those of simple sugars, and are more readily stored as fat, if not limited to following high-intensity exercise only. For health reasons, avoid foods containing high-fructose corn syrup.

4 ▶ *Eat fiber.* Fibrous carbohydrates include leafy green vegetables, broccoli, cauliflower, cucumbers, onions, peppers, and many other vegetables. Because fiber cannot be digested by the human GI tract, it is passed as waste. It is, nonetheless, vital to good health. Inadequate dietary fiber leads to a sluggish GI tract, water retention, bloating, constipation, and an increased risk of developing colon cancer. Although adequate dietary fiber is paramount to a healthy colon, it is calorically vacant. Hence, foods classified as fibrous carbohydrates can be eaten all day, in enormous quantities, without causing any weight gain. To ensure that you are consuming adequate fiber, include at least one serving of fresh fruit or vegetables with every meal.

5 ▶ *Include some fat with every meal.* Fats are important energy sources because stored glycogen is limited. Saturated fats may contribute to the development of CVD. Polyunsaturated and monounsaturated fats derived from plant sources are a healthier choice. Fat should comprise approximately 25 to 30 percent of your total caloric intake. Because fat causes you to feel satiated longer while stabilizing blood-sugar levels, it should be consumed with every meal. If your daily fare doesn't contain enough fat and you find you have to add fat to your diet, choose healthy plant sources such as nuts, seeds, olive oil, sesame oil, flaxseed oil, and avocado. Avoid fried foods, fatty sauces and gravy, butter, margarine, and processed meats.

6 ▶ *Stay hydrated!* Water aids the liver and kidneys in the detoxification of poisons and the elimination of wastes from the body. Without sufficient water, we become dehydrated, our organs (including muscles, liver, and kidneys) do not function optimally, and metabolism suffers.

7

The Javalution Fitness Program

The unprecedented *per capita* weight gain that has been observed in the United States over the last twenty years is mirrored by a startling decrease in physical activity among virtually every segment of the population, including young children. Just about every study ever done on the subject has consistently demonstrated that activity level is inversely proportional to fat gain. In fact, more than any other factor, exercise is commonly cited as the best predictor for long-term weight management.

EXERCISE 101:
EXERCISING FOR LOOKS AND LONGEVITY

Body composition aside, regular exercise is vital to good health. In fact, research indicates that obese men who are active and cardiovascularly fit are not only less likely to suffer from heart disease than lean men who are sedentary, they are also less likely to die of *any* cause than lean, sedentary men. A study looked at 21,925 men, aged thirty to eighty-three years, who had a body-composition assessment and a maximal treadmill exercise test. Interestingly, they discovered that unfit, lean men had a higher risk of all-cause and cardiovascular disease (CVD) mortality than did men who were fit and obese. The scientists concluded, "the health benefits of leanness are limited to fit men, and being fit may reduce the hazards of obesity."[1] Exercise appears to be extremely beneficial to overall health, even without weight loss, and it should come as no surprise that a sedentary lifestyle is one of the worst things you can do to your body.

Unfortunately, by the time most people are made aware that their body is suffering from the ravages of a sedentary lifestyle, it's too late to do much about it. Despite the dramatic increase in medical procedures to combat CVD, it remains the leading cause of death in the United States. According to the American Heart Association (AHA), more lives are lost to CVD every year than to cancer, accidents, Alzheimer's disease, and AIDS—*combined*. As it turns out, many of those fancy procedures for treating CVD have a very minimal effect on long-term survival. Like it or not, the only surefire way to "cure" heart disease remains to prevent it from happening in the first place.

Physical activity lowers cholesterol, blood pressure, and heart rate. In addition to its cardiovascular benefits, regular exercise decreases cancer risk and promotes bone health, gastrointestinal (GI) health, and even mental health. Those who exercise regularly are less depressed, suffer less anxiety, sleep better, and have more energy, higher self-esteem, and a better body image than sedentary individuals.

Despite the unambiguously pivotal role that regular exercise plays in good physical and mental health, the fact remains that one in four American adults is completely sedentary. Of those who exercise at all, 75 percent of us do not get enough exercise to positively affect our health. Half of all people who begin a new program of regular exercise will abandon it in less than twelve months. Why are the statistics so dismal? After all, we know that regular exercise will make us healthier, happier, and more energized. We know that regular exercise has a significant impact on both our quality of life and our overall longevity. In fact, most of us actually enjoy the process of exercising! As a nation of reasonably intelligent, well-informed individuals, why can't we stick to a simple workout schedule?

The number-one reason people cite for not exercising is lack of time. But when you realize that as little as twenty-five minutes of vigorous activity every other day can have a significant impact on your overall health and longevity, lack of time seems like a poor excuse. Many others find the notion of starting to exercise overwhelmingly intimidating. If you count yourself among them, you should be aware that if you've been sedentary for a prolonged period of time or if you are significantly overweight or obese, something as simple as walking is the perfect way to ease into a more active lifestyle. If you're one of the many unfortunates who keep falling off the exercise wagon because past attempts have not yielded the results you'd hoped for, you should know that there are many ways to increase the effectiveness of your training.

For optimal health and body composition, the American College of Sports Medicine currently recommends that all able-bodied individuals engage in a variety of physical activities which include twenty to sixty minutes of cardiovascular exercise three to five days a week, plus at least two weekly sessions of resistance and flexibility training.

So, get rid of your excuses, get moving, get lean, and get healthy!

LET'S GET STARTED

Before diving headfirst into a new exercise program, take a moment to familiarize yourself with the basics of safe, effective training. There are a handful of simple rules everyone should follow to exercise comfortably, minimize the risk of injury, and maximize training efficiency. Remember, the more you enjoy working out and the more satisfied you are with your training results, the easier it will be to make a lasting commitment to physical activity.

Rule number one: Never tax a cold muscle. Just like steel and concrete, our muscles, tendons, and ligaments possess material properties that react to heat and cold. A "cold" muscle feels stiff and weak, and compared to a warm muscle, it *is* stiff and weak. Similarly, a warm tendon or ligament will safely accommodate more stretch than a cold one. Before participating in any vigorous athletic activity, including stretching, running, or weight training, you should raise your peripheral body temperature. Get your heart beating and increase the blood flow to your extremities by participating in five minutes of a low-intensity cardiovascular activity. Try knee raises and windmills or hop on the stationary bike or treadmill at a low setting.

If you've been inactive for a prolonged period of time or if you are extremely overweight, walking is a great way to start getting fit. Although it does not impose the same high-impact stresses as running, it is still very important to invest in quality footwear that incorporates proper ankle support and a well-cushioned sole. Under your doctor's supervision, start with a reasonable goal, such as ten or fifteen minutes of brisk walking, five or six days a week. As your fitness level improves, work your way up to thirty to forty minutes, five or six days a week.

Even if you are already lean and moderately active, dramatically altering your current routine may render you temporarily vulnerable to injury. Whenever you significantly increase your activity level or take up a new sport, remember that you will be using your muscles and joints in unusual and untested ways. To minimize your risk of injury, always increase your activity level in reasonable increments of 5 to 10 percent per week, and ease gradually into new activities.

For example, if you're an avid swimmer and decide to take up running, the fact that your cardiovascular system may be extremely fit has nothing to do with it. You are subjecting your spine, hips, knees, and ankles to enormous amounts of new and different stimuli and stress with each stride. Any instability will contribute to microtrauma, pain, and inflammation. Before you undertake a vigorous running program, first work to strengthen the muscles and ligaments that stabilize your joints. You may want to start slowly by walking (not running) stairs and hills. After two to three weeks of conditioning, try running on a forgiving surface such as wood, dirt, sand, or grass. You should limit how often you run on concrete or asphalt, because the inflexibility of these hard surfaces will produce unhealthy stresses on every weight-bearing joint in your body.

CARDIO

Twenty to thirty minutes of moderate-intensity aerobic activity per day, either all at once or accumulated throughout the day, on most days of the week is the minimum requirement for good heart health. In the same amount of time it takes you to watch your favorite sitcom, taking a brisk walk will effectively combat just about every major risk factor for heart disease—including high blood pressure, high cholesterol, stress, obesity, diabetes, and atherosclerosis. By increasing your walking time or adding more vigorous exercise to your regimen, you reduce your risk even further. And as an added bonus, studies have shown that this amount of physical activity also reduces the risk of cancer.

The intensity of your cardio workouts should coincide with your training goals. If your primary goal is fat loss or weight maintenance, you might be surprised to learn that low- to moderate-intensity activities such as brisk walking, which causes your heart to beat at approximately 60 to 70 percent of your maximum heart rate, are actually ideal for fat burning.

To calculate your Target Aerobic Zone (TAZ), first subtract your age from the number 220 to estimate maximum heart rate (MHR). For fundamental cardiovascular health and fat burning, multiply this figure by 60 percent and by 70 percent. The two results generated represent the upper and lower limits of your TAZ in beats per minute (BPM). For example, a forty-year-old woman would have a TAZ of:

▶ **TARGET AEROBIC ZONE (TAZ)**

$$= (MHR) \times (0.60 \text{ to } 0.70) \text{ BPM}$$

$$= (220 - 40) \times (0.60 \text{ to } 0.70)$$

$$= (180 \times 0.60) \text{ to } (180 \times 0.70)$$

$$= 108 \text{ to } 126 \text{ BPM}$$

The simplest way to be sure that you are exercising within your targeted zone is to wear a heart-rate monitor. Once you learn what it "feels like" to exercise within your target zone, you may no longer need to consult your heart-rate monitor to achieve the desired results unless you are following a specific competition protocol. In the absence of a heart-rate monitor, a good rule of thumb for simple fat burning is to exercise at a pace where you can carry on a conversation with effort, but would find it impossible to whistle a tune.

RESISTANCE

Although weight training and other forms of resistance exercise cannot take the place of aerobic activity, a recent position paper published by the AHA indicates that mild- to moderate-resistance exercise is effective for decreasing major coronary-risk factors such as hypertension. Not only that, but studies show that a combination of cardiovascular and resistance training decreases the lean-tissue (muscle) loss that can result from dieting.

The more lean tissue, or muscle mass, you possess, the more calories you will burn all day, every day, regardless of your activity level. In essence, your muscle actually helps eat your fat stores! How does this miracle occur?

▶ First, contracting your muscles requires substantial caloric expenditure. Every time you train, you are burning calories.

▶ Second, exercise transiently raises your metabolic rate for several hours following each session. Hence, you continue to burn extra calories even if you're just lying on the couch watching TV.

▶ Third, studies have demonstrated that each pound of muscle you have requires approximately thirty-five calories per day just to exist. The more muscle you have, the higher your resting metabolic rate (RMR), and the greater your overall caloric expenditure.

The only way to reliably prevent the lean-tissue loss that accompanies aging is through regular resistance exercise such as weightlifting. The American College of Sports Medicine recommends two to three sessions of resistance exercise per week. Unfortunately, although it's not rocket science, weight training is an art that cannot be mastered overnight. For every correct way to perform an exercise, there are a dozen ways to do it wrong. Improper training techniques inevitably lead to injury, futile wasted hours, and an asymmetric physique.

We all know people who spend their life in the gym and never seem to make any progress. These individuals could probably benefit from a couple of sessions with a competent personal trainer. Whether you are a world-class athlete or a phys-ed flunky, whether you've just invested in your first gym membership or have been training for years, there are several basic tenets of weightlifting that apply to everyone. The following fundamentals are guaranteed to maximize your gains and efficiency while minimizing your risk of burnout and injury.

Train Your Entire Body

A well-designed training program addresses all of the major muscle groups. Full-body training prevents muscular imbalances that can lead to injury while it provides you with a well-proportioned, symmetrical appearance. Table 7.1 provides an example of a standard, novice workout (follow this routine two to three times per week).

TABLE 7.1. STANDARD NOVICE WORKOUT			
Target	Exercise	Sets	Reps
Abs	crunches	3	20–30
Biceps	seated dumbbell curls	3	15–20
Triceps	dumbbell kick backs	3	15–20
Shoulders	seated shoulder press	3	15–20
Pectorals	push-ups	3	AMAP*
Back	dumbbell rows	3	15–20
Calves	calf extensions	3	AMAP*
Thighs/Glutes	leg press	3	15–20

*as many as possible

Use Good Form

When learning to train with weights, movements must be accomplished with strict attention to form and technique. Hold the full contraction for a short pause to accentuate the pump. Concentrate on both the concentric (when the muscle is actively shortening) and the eccentric (when the muscle is actively lengthening) phases of the contraction to maximize every repetition. Be certain to exercise throughout the full range of motion. Learn what using specific muscle groups "feels like," and duplicate this feeling when trying new exercises for the same body part. Most importantly, avoid sharp, jerky repetitions and using momentum to lift a heavier weight.

Learn to Isolate

Steady, controlled movements are the key to learning what it "feels like" to work a specific muscle or muscle group. It takes about three weeks for the novice to maximize the neuromuscular coordination necessary to identify and fully recruit muscle fibers from individual muscle groups. After three weeks, you will be able to efficiently target these groups and minimize cheating with sympathetic muscles. You will also be able to use virtually any unfamiliar piece of gym equipment (and invent your own exercises) simply by duplicating the appropriate "feel" when trying a new exercise for the same body part.

Train within the Appropriate Range

The weight you lift must be heavy enough to challenge your muscles or you will make little progress. On the other hand, you should avoid extreme resistances, which put you at an increased risk for injury. How do you choose the correct weight for a particular exercise? If you're new to weightlifting, it's going to take a little trial and error. Start light and go for high reps (20–30 per set). As mentioned, it takes about three weeks for the novice to maximize the neuromuscular coordination necessary to identify and fully recruit muscle fibers from individual muscle groups. Then, you should gradually increase the intensity of your training by progressing to heavier weights and a lower rep range.

Gradual Progress for Safe Gains

Every strength-training program needs a protocol for safe, effective progress. Eventually, most people develop an intuitive sense of how and when they should increase their training intensity. Until that happens, use about 5 percent additional resistance whenever you are able to perform a given movement, with good form, for at least one repetition in excess of your target range for that exercise.

Mix It Up

Even the most brilliantly designed training program gradually loses its efficiency. In simple terms, your body is too smart for its own good. As you become more and more adept at performing a particular movement, the results produced by that particular movement will reach a plateau. It's time to mix things up. Your entire workout should be modified every few weeks for best results.

▶ Constantly try new exercises to add to your repertoire.

▶ Look around the gym.

▶ Talk to people.

▶ Consult magazines.

▶ Experiment on your own: Change bench angles, alter foot stances, switch the order of your exercises, try super sets, strip sets, and so on.

▶ Be creative!

Listen to Your Body

After bad form, overtraining is the most common mistake in the gym. If you find you are losing enthusiasm for your workouts, if you are constantly tired, or if your progress has slowed or stopped, it's time for a break. If you have been training consistently, take a week off every two to three months. You will return to the gym reinvigorated, renewed, and rested. You won't lose strength in one week. Even after a month off, chances are you will surprise yourself by returning to the gym stronger than when you left. Following a break is the ideal time to modify your training program.

Be Patient

You will see progress if you are patient and stick with it! No two physiques are exactly the same, and you should not measure your progress against others. Why don't you take some photos now and compare them to how you look three months from now? You will be amazed by the progress you've made.

8

Frequently Asked Questions

▶ *What's the lowdown on coffee? Is it good or bad for your health?*

According to the summary of a study published in 2005, scientists stated, "coffee is probably the most frequently ingested beverage worldwide; actually, we think water is . . . but who's arguing? Coffee is also a rich source of many other ingredients that may contribute to its biological activity, such as heterocyclic compounds that exhibit strong antioxidant activity. Based on the literature reviewed, it is apparent that moderate, daily, filtered-coffee intake is not associated with any adverse effects on cardiovascular outcome. On the contrary, the data shows that coffee has significant antioxidant activity, and may have an inverse association with the risk of type 2 diabetes."[1] In fact, coffee:

▶ Helps maintain testosterone levels in men.

▶ May lower the risk of Parkinson's disease.

▶ May lower the risk of gallstones.

▶ May lower the risk of type 2 diabetes.

▶ Has no effect on the incidence of heart disease.

▶ Has no association with breast cancer incidence.

▶ What is the real effect of coffee on blood pressure?

One study looked at the effect of decaffeinated versus regular (caffeinated) coffee on blood pressure and heart rate in a randomized, double-blind, crossover trial of forty-five healthy volunteers (twenty-three women and twenty-two men, aged twenty-five to forty-five years old) with a habitual intake of four to six cups of coffee/day. The subjects received five cups of regular coffee each day for a period of six weeks, and five cups of decaffeinated coffee every day for the next six weeks, or vice versa. The background diet was kept the same. The total amount of caffeine ingested was 40 milligrams (mg) during the decaffeinated coffee period and 445 mg during the regular coffee period. Use of decaffeinated coffee led to a significant but small decrease in systolic (down 1.5 millimeters [mm] of mercury [Hg]) and diastolic (down 1.0 mm Hg) ambulant blood pressure and to a small increase in ambulant heart rate (up 1.3 beats per minute). The authors of the study concluded that in "normotensive" adults (those with normal blood pressure), replacement of regular by decaffeinated coffee leads to a real but small drop in blood pressure.

Despite what these doctors have concluded, we must interject that a 1.0–1.5 mm Hg alteration in blood pressure is not clinically meaningful. If you go to your physician and have your blood pressure measured, it can vary by as much as 1–10 mm Hg from visit to visit. This study is an example of how "statistically significant" findings are in actuality "physiologically meaningless."[2] Furthermore, it should be noted that many large-scale studies show no long-term effect of coffee consumption on blood pressure.

Does coffee increase your risk of arthritis?

Scientists determined whether coffee, decaffeinated coffee, total coffee, tea, or overall caffeine consumption was associated with the risk of rheumatoid arthritis (RA) using the Nurses' Health Study, a longitudinal cohort study of 121,701 women. Accordingly, they found "little evidence of an association between coffee, decaffeinated coffee, or tea consumption and the risk of RA among women."[3]

Does drinking coffee with a meal further enhance the thermic or thermogenic effect (metabolic-rate enhancement) of the meal?

Yes! There are studies that show that the thermic effect of a meal is significantly greater after caffeinated coffee than after decaffeinated coffee and, again, fat oxidation is significantly greater after regular coffee. In conclusion, caffeinated coffee stimulates metabolic rate in both control and obese individuals; however, this increase is accompanied by greater fat oxidation in subjects of normal weight.[4]

Another study showed that the thermic effect of caffeinated and decaffeinated coffee ingested with a standard breakfast produced in eight healthy subjects indirect calorimetric results. A higher increase in the metabolic rate was observed after consuming the breakfast with caffeinated coffee than after breakfast with decaffeinated coffee.[5]

Do people who drink coffee have higher cholesterol levels than those who do not?

In general, people who drink coffee do not have higher cholesterol levels than noncoffee drinkers.

▶ Does coffee make you fat or keep you from losing fat?

There is no evidence whatsoever to support this claim. In fact, the primary active ingredient in coffee is caffeine. Caffeine is a lipolytic agent, as well as a potent ergogenic aid. If that makes you fat, then the Earth is flat and unicorns really do exist!

▶ I heard that green tea extract can be used as a supplement to increase metabolism and fight fat? Is that true?

Yes! In fact, a landmark study looked at twenty-four-hour energy expenditure in ten healthy men who underwent three different treatments: green tea extract (50 mg caffeine and 90 mg *Epigallocatechin gallate* [EGCG]), caffeine (50 mg), and placebo, which they ingested at breakfast, lunch, and dinner. They found that relative to the placebo, treatment with the green tea extract resulted in a significant increase in calories burned over twenty-four hours. According to the authors, "green tea has thermogenic properties and promotes fat oxidation beyond that explained by its caffeine content per se. The green tea extract may play a role in the control of body composition via sympathetic activation of thermogenesis, fat oxidation, or both."[6] Among the Javalution functional coffees, JavaFit Energy Extreme has the benefits of coffee combined with the extra thermogenic boost from green tea extract.

▶ Does consuming calcium also help in losing weight or fat?

Yes! A study from the journal *Obesity Research* supports this notion. Scientists performed a randomized, placebo-controlled trial for thirty-two obese adults. Patients were maintained for twenty-four weeks on balanced deficit diets (500 kcal/day deficit) and randomized to a standard diet (400 to

500 mg of dietary calcium/day supplemented with placebo), a high-calcium diet (standard diet supplemented with 800 mg of calcium/day), or high-dairy diet (1,200 to 1,300 mg of dietary calcium/day supplemented with placebo). What happened? Patients assigned to the standard diet lost 6 percent of their body weight, which was increased by 26 percent on the high-calcium diet and 70 percent on the high-dairy diet. Fat loss was similarly augmented by the high-calcium and high-dairy diets, by 38 percent and 64 percent, respectively. One really fascinating finding was that fat loss from the trunk region represented 19 percent of total fat loss on the low-calcium diet. This fraction increased to 50 percent and 66 percent on the high-calcium and high-dairy diets, respectively.

What does this mean? Keep in mind that truncal fat is bad; your body is basically a ticking timebomb waiting to die a sudden death from a heart attack. So, keep the beer belly to a minimum. Drink milk or take calcium. Better yet, drink JavaFit Lean with calcium.[7]

What is caffeine?

Chemists technically refer to caffeine as an alkaloid. There are several types of alkaloids of which caffeine belongs to a specific class called the "methylxanthines." Other methylxanthines include theophylline (used in medicines to treat asthma) and theobromine (found in chocolate). Each of these methylxanthines has stimulant properties.

How does caffeine itself taste?

Caffeine has a bitter taste.

What is a "moderate" intake of caffeine?

A moderate intake of caffeine for an adult is about 300 mg a day. That's roughly two to four cups of brewed coffee, or one to two cups of JavaFit Energy Extreme or JavaFit Burn Extreme. Different individuals have different tolerances to caffeine.

Why is caffeine added to so many medicines?

Because caffeine further enhances the analgesic (pain re-lieving) properties of medications. For instance, one study looked at the efficacy of a 100-mg diclofenac-sodium softgel (a non-steroidal anti-inflammatory [NSAID]) with or without 100 mg of caffeine versus placebo in individuals during migraine attacks. The major finding of the study was that the diclofenac softgel plus caffeine produced statistically signifi-cant benefits compared to the placebo at sixty minutes. The diclofenac softgel alone was no different than the placebo![8–10]

Another investigation looked at the benefits of acetamino-phen, aspirin, and caffeine (AAC) in the treatment of severe, disabling migraine attacks. Scientists concluded that "the non-prescription combination of AAC was well-tolerated and effective."[11–13] Perhaps this is one reason why caffeine helps exercise performance. You feel less pain during exercise and can therefore work out harder and with more intensity.

Is caffeine banned by the International Olympic Committee (IOC)?

Caffeine is no longer banned by the IOC. Nor is it banned by other sport-governing bodies (National Collegiate Athletic Association [NCAA], National Football League [NFL], Major League Baseball [MLB], National Basketball Association [NBA], the National Physique Committee [NPC], and the Interna-tional Federation of Bodybuilders [IFBB]).

What's an effective dose of caffeine to enhance exercise performance?

A range of 250–350 mg of caffeine seems to be sufficient to produce an ergogenic effect.

What's the best dose of caffeine to improve mental alertness and energy?

A range of 300–600 mg of caffeine is effective for enhancing energy.

What's the best dose of caffeine to promote fat burning and thermogenesis?

A range of 280–560 mg of caffeine will get your metabolic furnace turned up even higher!

Can you overdose on caffeine?

There are case reports of caffeine toxicity secondary to overdose. For instance, one individual ingested approximately 3.57 grams (g) of caffeine in a suicide attempt and developed rhabdomyolysis and acute renal failure. The patient was treated successfully. This case, according to the doctors, "represents a rarely reported complication of caffeine intoxication, rhabdomyolysis, which occurred in the absence of other toxins or conditions that predispose to muscle necrosis."[14]

There was another case of a twenty-year-old bulimic woman who ingested 20 g of caffeine in a suicide attempt. After being evaluated and discharged from the emergency department, she was readmitted with electrocardiogram (ECG) changes and ultimately found to have sustained a subendocardial infarction (a type of heart attack).

Keep in mind that these doses are more than eleven times greater than a typical daily serving of caffeine. Or to put it in perspective, in the first case, a 3.57 g dose of caffeine would be equal to 78 Diet Cokes and, in the second case, a 20 g dose would be equal to 438 Diet Cokes. The lethal dosage of caffeine that would reportedly kill 50 percent of the population (LD_50) is estimated by some to be 10 g for oral administration.

Should pregnant women avoid caffeine?

One study suggested that caffeine consumption may produce a small decrease in birth weight; however, it is "unlikely to be clinically important except for women consuming 600 mg [or more] of caffeine daily."[15] Another study looked at caffeine intake among 111 mothers of small-for-gestational-age (SGA) infants (fifty-six boys and fifty-five girls) compared to the intake among 747 mothers of non-SGA infants (368 boys and 379 girls). Mothers of SGA infants had a higher mean intake of caffeine [281 mg/day] in the third trimester than mothers of non-SGA infants (212 mg/day). Scientists concluded, "high caffeine intake in the third trimester may be a risk factor for fetal growth retardation, in particular if the fetus is a boy."[16] Also, a high intake of caffeine prior to pregnancy seems to be associated with an increased risk of spontaneous abortion, whereas low- to moderate-alcohol intake does not influence the risk.[17] The prudent course of action would be to limit caffeine consumption to less than 200 mg of caffeine daily. Certainly, it would be a good idea for pregnant women to seek their physician's advice.

What's the effect of caffeine on children?

Generally, caffeine is well-tolerated in the usual dietary amounts. There is evidence that individuals differ in their susceptibility to caffeine-related adverse effects, which in turn may influence their caffeine consumption. Overall, the effects of caffeine in children seem to be modest and typically innocuous.[18]

However, like any substance, there is a potential for abuse. One study reported on children and adolescents with daily or near-daily headaches and excessive consumption of caffeine in the form of cola drinks. The mean age of the subjects was 9.2 years (ranging from six to eighteen years), and the mean time of having daily or nearly daily headaches was 1.8 years (ranging from one-half year to five years). All were heavy cola consumers: at least 1.5 liters of cola drinks per day (192.88 mg of caffeine daily), and an average of 11 (ranging from 10.5–21) liters of cola drinks weekly, which amounts to 1,414.5 mg of caffeine (ranging from 1,350–2,700 mg). Patients were encouraged to achieve gradual withdrawal from cola drinks. Withdrawal led to complete cessation of all headaches in thirty-three subjects, whereas one boy and two adolescent girls continued to suffer from them.[19]

Based on the available evidence, scientists have concluded that children could consume up to 2.5 mg/kg of caffeine daily without troublesome effects. That's equal to 113 mg of caffeine for a 100-pound child.[20]

▶ Is caffeine addictive?

This isn't a trick question although you might think that folks use the word "addicted" in a rather reckless manner. Some liken caffeine "addiction" to a shopping "addiction" or a TV "addiction." Oddly enough, caffeine is not addictive by accepted definitions in the neuroscience literature. When regular caffeine consumption is abruptly ceased, some individuals may experience headache, fatigue, or drowsiness. Whether this qualifies as "addiction" in the strictest sense is debatable. According to a study published in the journal *Brain Research*, "low doses of caffeine, which reflect the usual human level of consumption, fail to activate reward circuits in the brain and thus provide functional evidence of the very low addictive potential of caffeine."[21]

Can caffeine increase the risk of heart disease?

Contrary to common belief, the published literature provides little evidence that coffee or caffeine in typical dosages increases the risk of heart attack, sudden death, or arrhythmia.[22] In one of the largest studies ever conducted, The Nurses' Health Study and Health Professionals' Follow-up Study, scientists followed 41,934 men from 1986 to 1998 and 84,276 women from 1980 to 1998. The participants did not have diabetes, cancer, or CVD at baseline. Coffee consumption was assessed every two to four years through validated questionnaires.

What did they discover? Scientists discovered an inverse association between coffee intake and type 2 diabetes after adjustment for age, body mass index (BMI), and other risk factors. Also, long-term coffee consumption is associated with a statistically significant lower risk for type 2 diabetes.[23] In other words, coffee or caffeine consumption may actually be good for you!

Another study indicated that consumers of high amounts of coffee have a reduced risk of type 2 diabetes and impaired glucose tolerance. The beneficial effects may involve both improved insulin sensitivity and enhanced insulin response.[24] However, if you are hypertensive or have several cardiovascular risk factors, it would be prudent for you to seek the advice of your doctor.

Does caffeine cause cancer?

There is no evidence that caffeine increases your risk of cancer. In the Swedish Mammography Screening Cohort, a large, population-based, prospective cohort study in Sweden comprised of 59,036 women aged forty to seventy-six years, scientists found that consumption of coffee, tea, and caffeine was not associated with breast cancer incidence.[25] In a case-control comparison of 323 women with benign breast disease and 1,458 controls, no differences were noted in the coffee and tea consumption patterns.[26] Even high-risk mice given caffeine showed an inhibition of tumor formation.[27]

▶ Does caffeine affect bone-mineral content in women?

Not if you add 1–2 tablespoons of milk to your coffee! The epidemiological studies showing a negative effect may be explained in part by an inverse relationship between consumption of milk and caffeine-containing beverages. In other words, low calcium intake per se, not consuming caffeinated beverages, is the main culprit. The negative effect of caffeine on calcium absorption is small enough to be fully offset by as little as 1–2 tablespoons of milk, according to a study published in 2002. There is no evidence that caffeine has any harmful effect on bone status or on calcium economy in individuals who ingest the currently recommended daily allowances of calcium.[28]

In a study of college-aged women, caffeine consumption was not associated with significant reduction in rates of bone gain. While calcium and protein nutrition affect bone gain in the third decade of life in women, moderate caffeine intake (one cup of coffee per day, or 103 mg) appears to be safe with respect to bone health in this age group.[29]

▶ How long does caffeine stay in your system?

The scientific term for how long something lasts in your body is "half-life." Half-life refers to the amount of time required for the potency of a drug or substance to fall to half of its original potency or to be eliminated from the body. For example, if the amount of a drug in your body is 10 of some measure with a half-life of two days, the amount left in your body after two days will be 5 of that original measure. Then, the amount drops by half each subsequent two days. In a study of normal-weight and obese subjects given 162 mg of caffeine orally, the half-life was slightly longer in obese (7.1 hours) versus normal-weight (5.4 hours) individuals.[30] Also, for women who use oral contraceptives, the half-life of caffeine tends to be longer (average of 7.9 hours versus 5.4 hours in the controls [women who don't take birth-control pills]).[31] In general, you could say that most normal-weight healthy individuals will eliminate 50 percent of the ingested caffeine from their body in five to six hours.

▶ How are JavaFit Burn Extreme and JavaFit Energy Extreme best used?

Consume JavaFit Burn Extreme or JavaFit Energy Extreme (two cups maximum) twenty to thirty minutes prior to exercise.

▶ How is JavaFit Lean with calcium best used?

Consume your typical serving of JavaFit Lean (two to four cups daily), plus make sure you eat plenty of dairy products (milk, low-fat cheese, and so on).

▶ What is Citrus aurantium (also known as "bitter orange")?

According to noted sports nutrition expert, Alan Shugarman, M.S., R.D., "*Citrus aurantium* is a citrus fruit that contains synephrine, N-methyltyramine, hordenine, tyramine, and octopamine. The active ingredients in bitter orange increase metabolism by stimulating the beta-3 receptors while not directly stimulating beta-1 and beta-2 receptors like ephedrine does. Compared to ephedrine, *Citrus aurantium* has little effect on heart rate and blood pressure. AdvantraZ™ is a brand of *Citrus aurantium* patented for thermogenesis (heat production), reducing body weight, and increasing lean muscle. The recommended dose is 60–120 mg per day in two to three doses. *Citrus aurantium* is often combined with caffeine to increase its effects on metabolism and calorie burning. You will often find *Citrus aurantium* in ephedrine-free weight-loss supplements. While research on the bitter orange for weight loss is not abundant, the product does show promise and more research is planned in the future."

▶ Can everyone consume Citrus aurantium?

If you are taking prescription medications or are nursing or pregnant, we recommend that you consult with a qualified health professional before consuming JavaFit Burn Extreme (which contains this herb).

▶ What is chromium?

It's a trace mineral that is involved in glucose (sugar) metabolism and the regulation of insulin levels.

▶ Is chromium supplementation safe?

Yes; most studies show no side effects. A few individuals may get an upset stomach.

▶ What is Garcinia cambogia?

Hydroxycitric acid (HCA) is the active ingredient extracted from this fruit. There is some animal data showing that HCA may suppress appetite. There are no adverse effects of HCA, although some individuals might get an upset stomach.

▶ Are the JavaFit coffee formulae patented?

Javalution has filed for patents to protect its proprietary blends.

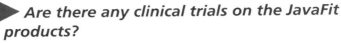

Are there any clinical trials on the JavaFit products?

Javalution has funded six different clinical trials. An initial pilot study performed by Dr. Ron Mendel of the Ohio Research Group showed that drinking two cups of JavaFit Burn Extreme could elevate your metabolic rate by a peak average of 25 percent! That's double the rate of regular coffee! There are also clinical trials ongoing at three major universities including Baylor University and the College of New Jersey. Javalution firmly believes that science lays the foundation for safe and effective high-quality products.

Welcome to the Javalution!

Not only can you derive the benefits of drinking coffee (which include a lower risk of type 2 diabetes and an energetic boost to your gray matter), but with the addition of nutraceuticals to coffee, the health- and fitness-promoting effects of coffee have now been enhanced. If you're a Starbucks drinker or a regular at your local convenience store, take the Javalution challenge. Drink one of the delicious JavaFit functional gourmet coffees and decide for yourself. If you're going to drink coffee, you might as well drink a delicious cup that's even better for you!

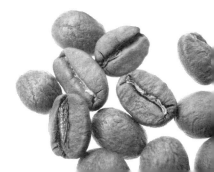

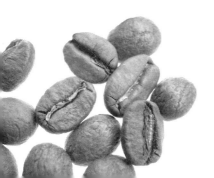

Fun Facts about Jose and Carla

Current Positions

▶ Chief Executive Officer of International Society of Sports Nutrition (ISSN)

▶ Chief Science Officer of Javalution

▶ Freelance Writer—*Muscular Development, Ironman, Max Sports Fitness,* and more

Birthplace

▶ Manila, Philippines

Education, Certifications, and Degress Attained

▶ B.S.—Biology, The American University, Washington, DC

▶ M.S.—Exercise Physiology, Kent State University

▶ Ph.D.—Muscle Physiology, University of Texas Southwestern Medical Center in Dallas

▶ Post-doctoral fellowship at University of Texas Southwestern

▶ Certified Strength and Conditioning Specialist

▶ Fellow of the American College of Sports Medicine

▶ Cofounder of the International Society of Sports Nutrition

▶ National Strength and Conditioning Association (NSCA) Research Achievement Award

Quick Fitness / Nutrition Tip

▶ Consume a "meal" immediately after each workout; your recovery will be much better!

Training Maxim

▶ Discipline is doing what's good for you even when you don't want to do it.

For Fun in My Spare Time

▶ Hanging out with my twin daughters, movies, dining out

Favorite Foods

▶ Sushi, Italian food (when in New York City!)

Most Frequently Watched Movie

▶ *Enter the Dragon*

Vacation Spot

▶ South Florida

CARLA SANCHEZ, C.S.C.S.

Current Positions

▶ Owner and Coach, The Performance Ready Fitness & Figure Team
▶ International Federation of Bodybuilders (IFBB) Pro Athlete
▶ Promoter, The Carla Sanchez Fitness Fiesta
▶ Writer, *Real Solutions* magazine
▶ Speaker, International Society of Sports Nutrition (ISSN)
▶ Fitness model
▶ NPC CO Trainer of the Year Award three times and Best of CO, Competitor of the Year in 1997

Birthplace

Colorado Springs, Colorado

Education, Certifications, and Degress Attained

▶ B.A.—Psychology, The Colorado College
▶ Certified Strength and Conditioning Specialist

Quick Fitness / Nutrition Tip

▶ Consume a serving of lean protein with every meal.

Training Maxim

▶ If you want serious results, take your training and diet seriously!

For Fun in My Spare Time

▶ Hanging out in bookstores, spa retreats, escaping to the mountains with my husband

Favorite Foods

▶ Mexican food, sushi, and peanut butter!

Most Frequently Watched Movie

▶ *Pulp Fiction*

Vacation Spot

▶ Mexico

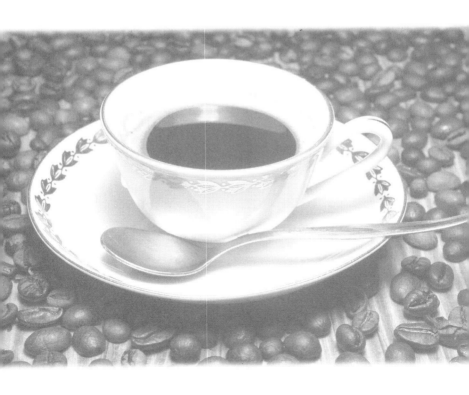

The Carla Sanchez Performance Ready Team

The Carla Sanchez Performance Ready (PR) Fitness & Figure Team—recognized as the finest fitness and figure competitors in the nation—was founded in August 2000 and boasts several of the nation's top fitness and figure athletes and fitness models. This group of diverse women, ranging in age from twenty to forty years, all share a common goal . . . to compete and become recognized as top national fitness/figure competitors. These women are truly committed to the pursuit of excellence and are driven to be the best in their sport.

Carla Sanchez, International Federation of Bodybuilders (IFBB) Pro Athlete and Certified Strength and Conditioning Specialist, coaches and advises each PR Team athlete through individualized training programs, diet planning, and precontest preparations, and leads team workouts, workshops, and seminars. Carla covers every detail to ensure a winning presentation on stage!

The PR Team trains together, shares helpful tips and competition experiences with one another, and offers support and encouragement to each other to promote individual success. As competitors, the PR Team athletes portray a striking balance of athleticism, beauty, power, and grace. They perform polished and skillful fitness routines, display strong and shapely physiques, and always present winning attitudes and exemplify their dedication to a fit and healthy lifestyle. Together they achieve success thanks to a cohesive team effort!

If you live in the state of Colorado and have always thought about competing in a Fitness or Figure competition, but didn't know where to begin, join Carla's PR Team! For more information visit www.performanceready.com or send an e-mail to Carla@carlasanchez.com.

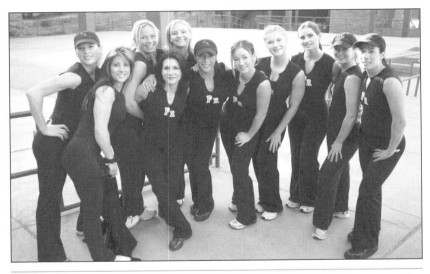

Members of the PR Team (from left to right): Sarah Gilbert, Christine Pomponio-Pate, Abbe Dorn, Jameela Klaimy, Carla Rae Weimer, Carla Sanchez, Shelly Howard, Jessie Booth, Brandy Newman, Jacqui Blazier, Judy Warren

Career highlights of a few of the nation's top competitors and fitness models from The Carla Sanchez Performance Ready Team:

Jacqui Blazier
- 2004 NPC Natural Colorado Fitness and Figure Championships—Class B Figure Champion

Jessie Booth
- 2004 NPC National Collegiate Figure Championships— Tall Class Champion
- 2004 NPC Natural Colorado Fitness and Figure Championships—Class C Figure Champion

Tanisha Harrison
- 2004 NPC National Figure Championships—Class E; seventh place
- 2003 NPC Jr. National Figure Championships—Class D; sixth place
- 2001 NPC Carol Semple Fitness and Figure Championships— Overall Figure Champion

Shelly Howard
- 2004 NPC Carol Semple Fitness and Figure Championships— Fitness Short Class; second place

Jameela Klaimy
- 2005 NPC Northern Colorado Fitness and Figure Championships—Class C Figure; second place

Brooke Paulin
- 2004 NPC National Fitness Championships—Medium Class; third place [first place Physique]
- 2004 NPC Colorado State Fitness and Figure Championships— Medium Class; first place in Fitness & Figure division
- 2004 NPC Orange County Classic—Overall Fitness Champion and first place Figure Medium Class

Christine Pomponio-Pate, IFBB Figure Pro
- 2005 IFBB San Francisco Pro Figure Championships; third place
- 2005 IFBB Figure International; fourth place
- 2004 IFBB Figure Olympia; sixth place
- 2004 IFBB GNC Show of Strength; fourth place
- 2004 IFBB NY Pro Figure Championships; second place
- 2004 IFBB California Pro Figure Championships; sixth place

Tara Richards
- 2004 NPC Orange County Classic—Class C Figure; second place

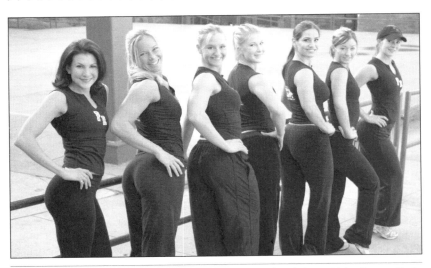

Members of the PR Team (from left to right): Jameela Klaimy, Abbe Dorn, Carla Rae Weimer, Jessie Booth, Brandy Newman, Shelly Howard, Jacqui Blazier

Ami Seier
- 2003 NPC Northern Colorado Fitness and Figure Championships—Tall Class Figure; third place

Judy Warren
- 2004 NPC Natural Colorado Fitness and Figure Championships—Class B Figure; second place

Carla Rae Weimer
- 2004 NPC USA Fitness Championships—eighth place
- 2004 NPC National Collegiate Figure Championships—Medium Class; second place
- 2004 NPC Colorado State Fitness and Figure Championships—Overall Fitness Champion and first place Figure Tall Class
- 2004 NPC Northern Colorado Fitness and Figure Championships—Fitness Short Class; first place and Figure Medium Class; second place

▶ **To meet the rest of the PR Team, visit www.performanceready. com.**

Notes and Additional References

Chapter 1

1. www.coffeeresearch.org/market/usa.htm.

2. Dulloo, A.G., C.A. Geissler, T. Horton, et al. "Normal caffeine consumption: influence on thermogenesis and daily energy expenditure in lean and postobese human volunteers." *The American Journal of Clinical Nutrition.* Jan 1989;49(1):44–50.

3. Acheson, K.J., B. Zahorska-Markiewicz, P. Pittet, et al. "Caffeine and coffee: their influence on metabolic rate and substrate utilization in normal weight and obese individuals." *The American Journal of Clinical Nutrition.* May 1980;33(5):989–997.

4. Jung, R.T., P.S. Shetty, W.P. James, et al. "Caffeine: its effect on catecholamines and metabolism in lean and obese humans." *Clinical Science (London).* May 1981;60(5):527–535.

5. Bracco, D., J.M. Ferrarra, M.J. Arnaud, et al. "Effects of caffeine on energy metabolism, heart rate, and methylxanthine metabolism in lean and obese women." *The American Journal of Physiology.* Oct 1995; 269(4 Pt 1):E671–678.

6. http://my.webmd.com/hw/drug_data/d04378a1?orgpath=/hw/drug_data/d04378a1#d04378a1-whatis

7. Costill, D.L., G.P. Dalsky, and W.J. Fink. "Effects of caffeine ingestion on metabolism and exercise performance." *Medicine and Science in Sports.* Fall 1978;10(3):155–158.

Chapter 2

1. Mendel, R.W., J.E. Hofheins, and T.N. Ziegenfuss. "Effect of JavaFit Extreme on Metabolic Rate, Substrate Utilization, and Cardiovascular Safety." International Society of Sports Nutrition. Abstract; 2004.

2. www.sportsnutritionsociety.org/site/admin/pdf/ISSN%20Abstracts%20SNRJ%201-1-S1-14-2004b.pdf

Chapter 3

1. Zahorska-Markiewicz, B. "The thermic effect of caffeinated and decaffeinated coffee ingested with breakfast." *Acta Physiologica Polonica.* Jan–Feb 1980;31(1):17–20.

2. Powers, S.K., and S. Dodd. "Caffeine and endurance performance." *Sports Medicine (Auckland, N.Z.).* May–Jun 1985;2(3):165–174.

3. Arciero, P.J., A.W. Gardner, J. Calles-Escandon, et al. "Effects of caffeine ingestion on NE kinetics, fat oxidation, and energy expenditure in younger and older men." *The American Journal of Physiology.* Jun 1995;268(6 Pt 1):E1192–1198.

4. Acheson, K.J., B. Zahorska-Markiewicz, P. Pittet, et al. "Caffeine and coffee: their influence on metabolic rate and substrate utilization in normal weight and obese individuals." *The American Journal of Clinical Nutrition.* May 1980;33(5):989–997.

5. Ryu, S., S.K. Choi, S.S. Joung, et al. "Caffeine as a lipolytic food component increases endurance performance in rats and athletes." *Journal of Nutritional Science and Vitaminology.* Apr 2001;47(2):139–146.

6. See Note 3.

Chapter 4

1. Hindmarch, I., U. Rigney, N. Stanley, et al. "A naturalistic investigation of the effects of day-long consumption of tea, coffee and water on alertness, sleep onset and sleep quality." *Psychopharmacology.* Apr 2000;149 (3):203–216.

2. Johnson-Kozlow, M., D. Kritz-Silverstein, E. Barrett-Connor, et al. "Coffee consumption and cognitive function among older adults." *American Journal of Epidemiology.* Nov 1 2002;156(9):842–850.

3. Paluska, S.A. "Caffeine and exercise." *Current Sports Medicine Reports.* Aug 2003;2(4):213–219.

4. McLellan, T.M., and D.G. Bell. "The impact of prior coffee consumption on the subsequent ergogenic effect of anhydrous caffeine." *International Journal of Sport Nutrition and Exercise Metabolism.* Dec 2004;14(6):698–708.

5. Cole, K.J., D.L. Costill, R.D. Starling, et al. "Effect of caffeine ingestion on perception of effort and subsequent work production." *International Journal of Sport Nutrition.* Mar 1996;6(1):14–23.

6. Wiles, J.D., S.R. Bird, J. Hopkins, et al. "Effect of caffeinated coffee on running speed, respiratory factors, blood lactate and perceived exertion during 1500-m treadmill running." *British Journal of Sports Nutrition.* Jun 1992;26(2):116–120.

7. Costill, D.L., G.P. Dalsky, and W.J. Fink. "Effects of caffeine ingestion on metabolism and exercise performance." *Medicine and Science in Sports.* Fall 1978;10(3):155–158.

8. Anderson, M.E., C.R. Bruce, S.F. Fraser, et al. "Improved 2000-meter rowing performance in competitive oarswomen after caffeine ingestion." *International Journal of Sport Nutrition and Exercise Metabolism.* Dec 2000;10(4):464–475.

9. Jacobson, B.H., M.D. Weber, L. Claypool, et al. "Effect of caffeine on maximal strength and power in elite male athletes." *British Journal of Sports Nutrition.* Dec 1992;26(4):276–280.

10. Collomp, K., S. Ahmaidi, J.C. Chatard, et al. "Benefits of caffeine ingestion on sprint performance in trained and untrained swimmers." *European Journal of Applied Physiology and Occupational Physiology.* 1992;64(4):377–380.

11. Strong, F.C., 3rd. "It may be the caffeine in Extra Strength Excedrin that is effective for migraine." *The Journal of Pharmacy and Pharmacology.* Dec 1997;49(12):1260.

12. www.headaches.org/consumer/educationalmodules/caffeine/fast. html

13. O'Connor, P.J., R.W. Motl, S.P. Broglio, et al. "Dose-dependent effect of caffeine on reducing leg muscle pain during cycling exercise is unrelated to systolic blood pressure." *Pain.* Jun 2004;109(3):291–298.

14. Motl, R.W., P.J. O'Connor, and R.K. Dishman. "Effect of caffeine on perceptions of leg muscle pain during moderate intensity cycling exercise." *The Journal of Pain: Official Journal of the American Pain Society.* Aug 2003;4(6):316–321.

15. Bell, D.G., and T.M. McLellan. "Exercise endurance 1, 3, and 6 h after caffeine ingestion in caffeine users and nonusers." *Journal of Applied Physiology.* Oct 2002;93(4):1227–1234.

16. Armstrong, L.E. "Caffeine, body fluid-electrolyte balance, and exercise performance." *International Journal of Sport Nutrition and Exercise Metabolism.* Jun 2002;12(2):189–206.

Chapter 5

1. Ranheim, T., and B. Halvorsen. "Coffee consumption and human health—beneficial or detrimental?—Mechanisms for effects of coffee consumption on different risk factors for cardiovascular disease and type 2 diabetes mellitus." *Molecular Nutrition & Food Research.* Feb 10 2005.

2. Yoshioka, K., A. Kogure, T. Yoshida, et al. "Coffee consumption and risk of type 2 diabetes mellitus." *Lancet.* Feb 22 2003;361(9358):703.

3. "Coffee linked to reduced risk of diabetes." *Mayo Clinic Women's Healthsource.* Jun 2004;8(6):3.

4. "Food choices may affect diabetes risk. Coffee and magnesium-rich foods may deflect diabetes, while red meat may promote it." *Health News* (*Waltham, Mass.*). Mar 2004;10(3):3.

5. Summaries for patients. "Coffee drinkers at lower risk for type 2 diabetes." *Annals of Internal Medicine.* Jan 6 2004;140(1):I17.

6. Agardh, E.E., S. Carlsson, A. Ahlbom, et al. "Coffee consumption, type 2 diabetes and impaired glucose tolerance in Swedish men and women." *Journal of Internal Medicine.* Jun 2004;255(6):645–652.

7. Carlsson, S., N. Hammar, V. Grill, et al. "Coffee consumption and risk of type 2 diabetes in Finnish twins." *International Journal of Epidemiology.* Jun 2004;33(3):616–617.

8. Gerber, D.A. "Coffee consumption and type 2 diabetes mellitus." *Annals of Internal Medicine.* Aug 17 2004;141(4):323; author reply 323–324.

9. Glaser, J.H., and S.K. Glaser. "Coffee consumption and type 2 diabetes mellitus." *Annals of Internal Medicine.* Aug 17 2004;141(4):323; author reply 323-324.

10. Isogawa, A., M. Noda, Y. Takahashi, et al. "Coffee consumption and risk of type 2 diabetes mellitus." *Lancet.* Feb 22 2003;361(9358):703–704.

11. Louria, D.B. "Coffee consumption and type 2 diabetes mellitus." *Annals of Internal Medicine.* Aug 17 2004;141(4):321; author reply 323–324.

12. Reunanen, A., M. Heliovaara, and K. Aho. "Coffee consumption and risk of type 2 diabetes mellitus." *Lancet.* Feb 22 2003;361(9358):702–703; author reply 703.

13. Rosengren, A., A. Dotevall, L. Wilhelmsen, et al. "Coffee and incidence of diabetes in Swedish women: a prospective 18-year follow-up study." *Journal of Internal Medicine.* Jan 2004;255(1):89–95.

14. Salazar-Martinez, E., W.C. Willett, A. Ascherio, et al. "Coffee consumption and risk for type 2 diabetes mellitus." *Annals of Internal Medicine.* Jan 6 2004;140(1):1–8.

15. Saremi, A., M. Tulloch-Reid, and W.C. Knowler. "Coffee consumption and the incidence of type 2 diabetes." *Diabetes Care.* Jul 2003;26(7): 2211–2212.

16. Schaefer, B. "Coffee consumption and type 2 diabetes mellitus." *Annals of Internal Medicine.* Aug 17 2004;141(4):321; author reply 323–324.

17. Soriguer, F., G. Rojo-Martinez, and I.E. de Antonio. "Coffee consumption and type 2 diabetes mellitus." *Annals of Internal Medicine.* Aug 17 2004;141(4):321–323; author reply 323–324.

18. Tan, D.S. "Coffee consumption and risk of type 2 diabetes mellitus." *Lancet.* Feb 22 2003;361(9358):702; author reply 703.

19. Tuomilehto, J., G. Hu, S. Bidel, et al. "Coffee consumption and risk of type 2 diabetes mellitus among middle-aged Finnish men and women." *JAMA.* Mar 10 2004;291(10):1213–1219.

20. van Dam, R.M., and E.J. Feskens. "Coffee consumption and risk of type 2 diabetes mellitus." *Lancet.* Nov 9 2002;360(9344):1477–1478.

21. See Note 7.

22. See Note 13.

23. See Note 14.

24. See Note 19.

25. See Note 20.

26. van Dam, R.M., W.J. Pasman, and P. Verhoef. "Effects of coffee consumption on fasting blood glucose and insulin concentrations: randomized controlled trials in healthy volunteers." *Diabetes Care.* Dec 2004;27(12): 2990–2992.

27. Willett, W.C., M.J. Stampfer, J.E. Manson, et al. "Coffee consumption

and coronary heart disease in women. A ten-year follow-up." *JAMA.* Feb 14 1996;275(6):458–462.

28. See Note 13.

29. See Note 14.

30. Hogan, P., T. Dall, and P. Nikolov. "Economic costs of diabetes in the US in 2002." *Diabetes Care.* Mar 2003;26(3):917–932.

31. See Note 30.

32. Tavani, A., M. Bertuzzi, R. Talamini, et al. "Coffee and tea intake and risk of oral, pharyngeal and esophageal cancer." *Oral Oncology.* Oct 2003;39(7):695–700.

33. Kurozawa, Y., I. Ogimoto, A. Shibata, et al. "Dietary habits and risk of death due to hepatocellular carcinoma in a large scale cohort study in Japan. Univariate analysis of JACC study data." *The Kurume Medical Journal.* 2004;51(2):141–149.

34. http://story.news.yahoo.com/news?tmpl=story&u=/ap/20050216/ap_on_he_me/coffee_cancer; Feb 16 2005.

35. Jordan, S.J., D.M. Purdie, A.C. Green, et al. "Coffee, tea and caffeine and risk of epithelial ovarian cancer." *Cancer Causes & Control.* May 2004; 15(4):359–365.

36. Woolcott, C.G., W.D. King, and L.D. Marrett. "Coffee and tea consumption and cancers of the bladder, colon and rectum." *European Journal of Cancer Prevention.* Apr 2002;11(2):137–145.

37. Michels, K.B., L. Holmberg, L. Bergkvist, et al. "Coffee, tea, and caffeine consumption and breast cancer incidence in a cohort of Swedish women." *Annals of Epidemiology.* Jan 2002;12(1):21–26.

38. Michaud, D.S., E. Giovannucci, W.C. Willett, et al. "Coffee and alcohol consumption and the risk of pancreatic cancer in two prospective United States cohorts." *Cancer Epidemiology, Biomarkers & Prevention.* May 2001;10(5):429–437.

39. Gensini, G.F., and A.A. Conti. "[Does coffee consumption represent a coronary risk factor?]" *Recenti Progressi in Medicina.* Dec 2004;95(12): 563–565.

40. Basile, J. "Coffee intake over 33 years is not associated with developing hypertension." *Journal of Clinical Hypertension* (*Greenwich, Conn.*). Nov–Dec 2002;4(6):434.

41. Mukamal, K.J., M. Maclure, J.E. Muller, et al. "Caffeinated coffee consumption and mortality after acute myocardial infarction." *American Heart Journal.* Jun 2004;147(6):999–1004.

42. Jazbec, A., D. Simic, N. Corovic, et al. "Impact of coffee and other selected factors on general mortality and mortality due to cardiovascular disease in Croatia." *Journal of Health, Population, and Nutrition.* Dec 2003; 21(4):332–340.

43. See Note 27.

44. Kleemola, P., P. Jousilahti, P. Pietinen, et al. "Coffee consumption and the risk of coronary heart disease and death." *Archives of Internal Medicine.* Dec 11–25 2000;160(22):3393–3400.

45. Wakabayashi, K., S. Kono, K. Shinchi, et al. "Habitual coffee consumption and blood pressure: A study of self-defense officials in Japan." *European Journal of Epidemiology.* Oct 1998;14(7):669–673.

46. Lancaster, T., J. Muir, and C. Silagy. "The effects of coffee on serum lipids and blood pressure in a UK population." *Journal of the Royal Society of Medicine.* Sep 1994;87(9):506–507.

47. Rakic, V., V. Burke, and L.J. Beilin. "Effects of coffee on ambulatory blood pressure in older men and women: A randomized controlled trial." *Hypertension.* Mar 1999;33(3):869–873.

48. Hakim, A.A., G.W. Ross, J.D. Curb, et al. "Coffee consumption in hypertensive men in older middle-age and the risk of stroke: the Honolulu Heart Program." *Journal of Clinical Epidemiology.* Jun 1998;51(6):487–494.

Chapter 6

1. Berneis, K., R. Ninnis, D. Haussinger, et al. "Effects of hyper- and hypoosmolality on whole body protein and glucose kinetics in humans." *The American Journal of Physiology.* Jan 1999;276(1 Pt 1):E188–195.

2. Lemon, P.W. "Protein and amino acid needs of the strength athlete." *International Journal of Sport Nutrition.* Jun 1991;1(2):127–145.

3. Lemon, P.W., and D.N. Proctor. "Protein intake and athletic performance." *Sports Medicine* (*Auckland, N.Z.*). Nov 1991;12(5):313–325.

4. Phillips, S.M., J.W. Hartman, and S.B. Wilkinson. "Dietary protein to support anabolism with resistance exercise in young men." *Journal of the American College of Nutrition.* Apr 2005;24(2):134S–139S.

5. Poortmans, J.R., and O. Dellalieux. "Do regular high protein diets have potential health risks on kidney function in athletes?" *International Journal of Sport Nutrition and Exercise Metabolism.* Mar 2000;10(1):28–38.

6. Kerstetter, J.E., K.O. O'Brien, and K.L. Insogna. "Low protein intake: the impact on calcium and bone homeostasis in humans." *The Journal of Nutrition.* Mar 2003;133(3):855S–861S.

7. Kerstetter, J.E., K.O. O'Brien, and K.L. Insogna. "Dietary protein, calcium metabolism, and skeletal homeostasis revisited." *The American Journal of Clinical Nutrition.* Sep 2003;78(3 Suppl):584S–592S.

8. Heaney, R.P. "Is the paradigm shifting?" *Bone.* Oct 2003;33(4):457–465.

9. Kerstetter, J.E., K. O'Brien, and K. Insogna. "Dietary protein and intestinal calcium absorption." *The American Journal of Clinical Nutrition.* May 2001;73(5):990–992.

10. Heaney, R.P. "Protein intake and bone health: the influence of belief systems on the conduct of nutritional science." *The American Journal of Clinical Nutrition.* Jan 2001;73(1):5–6.

11. Heaney, R.P. "Factors influencing the measurement of bioavailability, taking calcium as a model." *The Journal of Nutrition.* Apr 2001;131(4 Suppl): 1344S–1348S.

12. Heaney, R.P. "Calcium needs of the elderly to reduce fracture risk." *Journal of the American College of Nutrition.* Apr 2001;20(2 Suppl):192S–197S.

13. Ruf, J.C. "Overview of epidemiological studies on wine, health and mortality." *Drugs Under Experimental and Clinical Research.* 2003;29(5-6):173–179.

14. Yancy, W.S., Jr., M.K. Olsen, J.R. Guyton, et al. "A low-carbohydrate, ketogenic diet versus a low-fat diet to treat obesity and hyperlipidemia: a randomized, controlled trial." *Annals of Internal Medicine.* May 18 2004; 140(10):769–777.

15. Weinberg, S.L. "The diet-heart hypothesis: a critique." *Journal of the American College of Cardiology.* Mar 3 2004;43(5):731–733.

16. Volek, J.S., M.J. Sharman, A.L. Gomez, et al. "Comparison of energy-restricted very low-carbohydrate and low-fat diets on weight loss and body composition in overweight men and women." *Nutrition & Metabolism.* Nov 8 2004;1(1):13.

17. Veech, R.L. "The therapeutic implications of ketone bodies: the effects

of ketone bodies in pathological conditions: ketosis, ketogenic diet, redox states, insulin resistance, and mitochondrial metabolism." *Prostaglandins, Leukotrienes, and Essential Fatty Acids.* Mar 2004;70(3):309–319.

18. Phinney, S.D. "Ketogenic diets and physical performance." *Nutrition & Metabolism.* Aug 17 2004;1(1):2.

19. Murray, A.J., R.E. Anderson, G.C. Watson, et al. "Uncoupling proteins in human heart." *Lancet.* Nov 13 2004;364(9447):1786–1788.

20. Layman, D.K., and J.I. Baum. "Dietary protein impact on glycemic control during weight loss." *The Journal of Nutrition.* Apr 2004;134(4): 968S–973S.

21. Feinman, R.D., and E.J. Fine. " 'A calorie is a calorie' violates the second law of thermodynamics." *Nutrition Journal.* Jul 28 2004;3(1):9.

22. Buchholz, A.C., C.F. McGillivray, and P.B. Pencharz. "Differences in resting metabolic rate between paraplegic and able-bodied subjects are explained by differences in body composition." *The American Journal of Clinical Nutrition.* Feb 2003;77(2):371–378.

23. Byrne, H.K., and J.H. Wilmore. "The effects of a 20-week exercise training program on resting metabolic rate in previously sedentary, moderately obese women." *International Journal of Sport Nutrition and Exercise Metabolism.* Mar 2001;11(1):15–31.

24. www.fda.gov/fdac/features/2003/503_fats.html

25. Clifton, P.M., J.B. Keogh, and M. Noakes. "Trans fatty acids in adipose tissue and the food supply are associated with myocardial infarction." *The Journal of Nutrition.* Apr 2004;134(4):874–879.

26. Oster, G., and D. Thompson. "Estimated effects of reducing dietary saturated fat intake on the incidence and costs of coronary heart disease in the United States." *Journal of the American Dietetic Association.* Feb 1996;96(2): 127–131.

27. Muller, H., A.S. Lindman, A.L. Brantsaeter, et al. "The serum LDL/HDL cholesterol ratio is influenced more favorably by exchanging saturated with unsaturated fat than by reducing saturated fat in the diet of women." *The Journal of Nutrition.* Jan 2003;133(1):78–83.

28. Sidhu, K.S. "Health benefits and potential risks related to consumption of fish or fish oil." *Regulatory Toxicology and Pharmacology: RTP.* Dec 2003;38(3):336–344.

29. See Note 28.

30. See Note 14.

31. Brehm, B.J., R.J. Seeley, S.R. Daniels, et al. "A randomized trial comparing a very low carbohydrate diet and a calorie-restricted low fat diet on body weight and cardiovascular risk factors in healthy women." *The Journal of Clinical Endocrinology and Metabolism.* Apr 2003;88(4):1617–1623.

32. Volek, J.S., M.J. Sharman, D.M. Love, et al. "Body composition and hormonal responses to a carbohydrate-restricted diet." *Metabolism: Clinical and Experimental.* Jul 2002;51(7):864–870.

33. See Note 21.

34. Johnston, C.S., C.S. Day, and P.D. Swan. "Postprandial thermogenesis is increased 100% on a high-protein, low-fat diet versus a high-carbohydrate, low-fat diet in healthy, young women." *Journal of the American College of Nutrition.* Feb 2002;21(1):55–61.

Chapter 7

1. Lee, C.D., S.N. Blair, and A.S. Jackson. "Cardiorespiratory fitness, body composition, and all-cause and cardiovascular disease mortality in men." *The American Journal of Clinical Nutrition.* Mar 1999;69(3):373–380.

Chapter 8

1. Ranheim, T., and B. Halvorsen. "Coffee consumption and human health—beneficial or detrimental?—Mechanisms for effects of coffee consumption on different risk factors for cardiovascular disease and type 2 diabetes mellitus." *Molecular Nutrition & Food Research.* Feb 10 2005.

2. van Dusseldorp, M., P. Smits, T. Thien, et al. "Effect of decaffeinated versus regular coffee on blood pressure. A 12-week, double-blind trial." *Hypertension.* Nov 1989;14(5):563–569.

3. Karlson, E.W., L.A. Mandl, G.N. Aweh, et al. "Coffee consumption and risk of rheumatoid arthritis." *Arthritis and Rheumatism.* Nov 2003;48(11):3055–3060.

4. Acheson, K.J., B. Zahorska-Markiewicz, P. Pittet, et al. "Caffeine and coffee: their influence on metabolic rate and substrate utilization in normal weight and obese individuals." *The American Journal of Clinical Nutrition.* May 1980;33(5):989–997.

5. Zahorska-Markiewicz, B. "The thermic effect of caffeinated and decaffeinated coffee ingested with breakfast." *Acta Physiologica Polonica.* Jan–Feb 1980;31(1):17–20.

6. Dulloo, A.G., C. Duret, D. Rohrer, et al. "Efficacy of a green tea extract rich in catechin polyphenols and caffeine in increasing 24-h energy expenditure and fat oxidation in humans." *The American Journal of Clinical Nutrition.* Dec 1999;70(6):1040–1045.

7. Zemel, M.B., W. Thompson, A. Milstead, et al. "Calcium and dairy acceleration of weight and fat loss during energy restriction in obese adults." *Obesity Research.* Apr 2004;12(4):582–590.

8. Forbes, J.A., K.F. Jones, C.J. Kehm, et al. "Evaluation of aspirin, caffeine, and their combination in postoperative oral surgery pain." *Pharmacotherapy.* 1990;10(6):387–393.

9. Goldstein, J., H.D. Hoffman, J.J. Armellino, et al. "Treatment of severe, disabling migraine attacks in an over-the-counter population of migraine sufferers: results from three randomized, placebo-controlled studies of the combination of acetaminophen, aspirin, and caffeine." *Cephalalgia.* Sep 1999;19(7):684–691.

10. Peroutka, S.J., J.A. Lyon, J. Swarbrick, et al. "Efficacy of diclofenac sodium softgel 100 mg with or without caffeine 100 mg in migraine without aura: a randomized, double-blind, crossover study." *Headache.* Feb 2004;44(2):136–141.

11. See Note 8.

12. See Note 9.

13. See Note 10.

14. Wrenn, K.D., and I. Oschner. "Rhabdomyolysis induced by a caffeine overdose." *Annals of Emergency Medicine.* Jan 1989;18(1):94–97.

15. Bracken, M.B., E.W. Triche, K. Belanger, et al. "Association of maternal caffeine consumption with decrements in fetal growth." *American Journal of Epidemiology.* Mar 1 2003;157(5):456–466.

16. Vik, T., L.S. Bakketeig, K.U. Trygg, et al. "High caffeine consumption in the third trimester of pregnancy: gender-specific effects on fetal growth." *Paediatric and Perinatal Epidemiology.* Oct 2003;17(4):324–331.

17. Tolstrup, J.S., S.K. Kjaer, C. Munk, et al. "Does caffeine and alcohol

intake before pregnancy predict the occurrence of spontaneous abortion?" *Human Reproduction (Oxford, England)*. Dec 2003;18(12):2704–2710.

18. Castellanos, F.X., and J.L. Rapoport. "Effects of caffeine on development and behavior in infancy and childhood: a review of the published literature." *Food and Chemical Toxicology*. Sep 2002;40(9):1235–1242.

19. Hering-Hanit, R., and N. Gadoth. "Caffeine-induced headache in children and adolescents." *Cephalalgia*. Jun 2003;23(5):332–335.

20. Nawrot, P., S. Jordan, J. Eastwood, et al. "Effects of caffeine on human health." *Food Additives and Contaminants*. Jan 2003;20(1):1–30.

21. Nehlig, A., and S. Boyet. "Dose-response study of caffeine effects on cerebral functional activity with a specific focus on dependence." *Brain Research*. Mar 6 2000;858(1):71–77.

22. Chou, T.M., and N.L. Benowitz. "Caffeine and coffee: effects on health and cardiovascular disease." *Comparative Biochemistry and Physiology. Part C, Pharmacology, Toxicology & Endocrinology*. Oct 1994;109(2):173–189.

23. Salazar-Martinez, E., W.C. Willett, A. Ascherio, et al. "Coffee consumption and risk for type 2 diabetes mellitus." *Annals of Internal Medicine*. Jan 6 2004;140(1):1–8.

24. Agardh, E.E., S. Carlsson, A. Ahlbom, et al. "Coffee consumption, type 2 diabetes and impaired glucose tolerance in Swedish men and women." *Journal of Internal Medicine*. Jun 2004;255(6):645–652.

25. Michels, K.B., L. Holmberg, L. Bergkvist, et al. "Coffee, tea, and caffeine consumption and breast cancer incidence in a cohort of Swedish women." *Annals of Epidemiology*. Jan 2002;12(1):21–26.

26. Marshall, J., S. Graham, and M. Swanson. "Caffeine consumption and benign breast disease: a case-control comparison." *American Journal of Public Health*. Jun 1982;72(6):610–612.

27. Lou, Y.R., Y.P. Lu, J.G. Xie, et al. "Effects of oral administration of tea, decaffeinated tea, and caffeine on the formation and growth of tumors in high-risk SKH-1 mice previously treated with ultraviolet B light." *Nutrition and Cancer*. 1999;33(2):146–153.

28. Heaney, R.P. "Effects of caffeine on bone and the calcium economy." *Food and Chemical Toxicology*. Sep 2002;40(9):1263–1270.

29. Packard, P.T., and R.R. Recker. "Caffeine does not affect the rate of gain in spine bone in young women." *Osteoporosis International*. 1996;6(2):149–152.

30. Abernethy, D.R., E.L. Todd, and J.B. Schwartz. "Caffeine disposition in obesity." *British Journal of Clinical Pharmacology.* Jul 1985;20(1):61–66.

31. Abernethy, D.R., and E.L. Todd. "Impairment of caffeine clearance by chronic use of low-dose oestrogen-containing oral contraceptives." *European Journal of Clinical Pharmacology.* 1985;28(4):425–428.

ADDITIONAL REFERENCES

Chapter 6

Agus, Michael S.D., Janis F. Swain, Courtney L. Larson, et al. "Dietary composition and physiologic adaptations to energy restriction." *The American Journal of Clinical Nutrition,* Vol. 71, No. 4, 901–907, April 2000.

Buchholz, A.C., and D.A. Schoeller. "Is a calorie a calorie?" *The American Journal of Clinical Nutrition.* 2004 May;79(5):899S–906S.

Butterfield, G.E. "Whole-body protein utilization in humans." *Medicine and Science in Sports and Exercise.* 1987 19:S157–S165.

Hedley, Allison A., PhD, Cynthia L. Ogden, PhD, Clifford L. Johnson, MSPH, et al. "Prevalence of overweight and obesity among U.S. children, adolescents, and adults, 1999-2002." *JAMA.* 2004;291:2847–2850.

Johnston, C.S., S.L. Tjonn, and P.D. Swan. "High-protein, low-fat diets are effective for weight loss and favorably alter biomarkers in healthy adults." *The Journal of Nutrition.* 2004 Mar;134(3):586–591.

Lemon, P.W.R. "Factors which appear to effect dietary protein need." *Journal of the American College of Nutrition,* Vol. 19, No. 90005, 513S–521S (2000).

Stanko, R.T., D.L. Tietze, and J.E. Arch. "Body composition, nitrogen metabolism, and energy utilization with feeding of mildly restricted (4.2 MJ/D) and severely restricted (2.1 MJ/D) isonitrogenous diets." *The American Journal of Clinical Nutrition.* 1992 Oct;56(4):636–640.

Chapter 7

Andersen, R.E., C.J. Crespo, S.J. Bartlett, et al. "Relationship of physical activity and television watching with body weight and level of fatness among children: results from the Third National Health and Nutrition Examination Survey." *JAMA.* 1998;279(12):938–942.

Andersen, R.E., Ph.D. "Exercise, an Active Lifestyle, and Obesity." *The Physician and Sportsmedicine.* 1999;(10).

Andersen, R.E., S.N. Blair, L.J. Cheskin, et al. "Encouraging patients to become more physically active: the physician's role." *Annals of Internal Medicine.* 1997;127(5):395–400.

Armstrong, K., and H. Edwards. "The effectiveness of a pram-walking exercise programme in reducing depressive symptomatology for postnatal women." *International Journal of Nursing Practice.* 2004 Aug;10(4):177–194.

Ballor, D.L., and E.T. Poehlman. "A meta-analysis of the effects of exercise and/or dietary restriction on resting metabolic rate." *European Journal of Applied Physiology.* 1995;71(6):535–542.

Lee, C.D., S.N. Blair, and A.S. Jackson. "Cardiorespiratory fitness, body composition, and all-cause and cardiovascular disease mortality in men." *The American Journal of Clinical Nutrition.* 1999;69(3):373–380.

Paluska, S.A., and T.L. Schwenk. "Physical activity and mental health: current concepts." *Sports Medicine (Auckland, N.Z.).* 2000 Mar;29(3):167–180.

Pollock, M.L., B.A. Franklin, G.J. Balady, et al. "Resistance exercise in individuals with and without cardiovascular disease: benefits, rationale, safety, and prescription: an advisory from the committee on exercise, rehabilitation, and prevention." Council on Clinical Cardiology, American Heart Association. *Circulation.* 2000;101(7):828–833.

Pollock, M.L., G.A. Gaesser, J.D. Butcher, et al. "The recommended quantity and quality of exercise for developing and maintaining cardiorespiratory and muscular fitness, and flexibility in healthy adults." *Medicine and Science in Sports and Exercise.* 1998;30(6):975–991.

U.S. Department of Health and Human Services. "Physical Activity and Health: A Report of the Surgeon General, Atlanta, DHHS." Centers for Disease Control and Prevention, National Center for Chronic Disease Prevention and Health Promotion, 1996.

Index